..pology of Contemporary Issues

A SERIES EDITED BY

ROGER SANJEK

Farm Work and Fieldwork: American Agriculture in Anthropological Perspective
EDITED BY MICHAEL CHIBNIK
The Varieties of Ethnic Experience: Kinship, Class, and Gender among California Italian-Americans
BY MICAELA DI LEONARDO
Lord I'm Coming Home: Everyday Aesthetics in Tidewater North Carolina
BY JOHN FORREST
Chinese Working-Class Lives: Getting By in Taiwan
BY HILL GATES
Accommodation without Assimilation: Sikh Immigrants in an American High School
BY MARGARET A. GIBSON
Praying for Justice: Faith, Order, and Community in an American Town
BY CAROL J. GREENHOUSE
Rx Spiritist as Needed: A Study of a Puerto Rican Community Mental Health Resource
BY ALAN HARWOOD
Between Two Worlds: Ethnographic Essays on American Jewry
EDITED BY JACK KUGELMASS
American Odyssey: Haitians in New York
BY MICHEL S. LAGUERRE
From Working Daughters to Working Mothers: Immigrant Women in a New England Industrial Community
BY LOUISE LAMPHERE
State and Family in Singapore: Restructuring an Industrial Society
BY JANET W. SALAFF
Uneasy Endings: Daily Life in an American Nursing Home
BY RENÉE ROSE SHIELD
Children of Circumstances: Israeli Emigrants in New York
BY MOSHE SHOKEID
City of Green Benches: Growing Old in a New Downtown
BY MARIA D. VESPERI
Renunciation and Reformulation: A Study of Conversion in an American Sect
BY HARRIET WHITEHEAD
Upscaling Downtown: Stalled Gentrification in Washington, D.C.
BY BRETT WILLIAMS
Women's Work and Chicano Families: Cannery Workers of the Santa Clara Valley
BY PATRICIA ZAVELLA

Uneasy Endings

DAILY LIFE IN AN
AMERICAN NURSING HOME

Renée Rose Shield

Cornell University Press

Ithaca and London

Copyright © 1988 by Renée Rose Shield

All rights reserved. Except for brief quotations in a review, this book, or parts thereof, must not be reproduced in any form without permission in writing from the publisher. For information, address Cornell University Press, 124 Roberts Place, Ithaca, New York 14850.

First published 1988 by Cornell University Press.

International Standard Book Number (cloth) 0-8014-2159-4
International Standard Book Number (paper) 0-8014-9490-7
Library of Congress Catalog Number 88-47743

Printed in the United States of America

Librarians: Library of Congress cataloging information appears on the last page of the book.

The paper in this book is acid-free and meets the guidelines for permanence and durability of the Committee on Production Guidelines for Book Longevity of the Council on Library Resources.

To Priscilla, who works here,
and to Sarah, who lives here

Contents

Preface   xi

Notebook: The 7:00 A.M. to 3:00 P.M. Shift   1

1. Anthropology in an American Nursing Home   10

Voice: Stanley Fierstein   25

2. Background and Context   28

Voice: Max Sager   38

3. Residents   42

Notebook: Resident-Care Conference   61

4. Conflicting Worldviews: Home versus Hospital   65

Notebook: Physical Therapy   80

Notebook: The Threatened Strike   86

5. The Total Institution   91

Notebook: 5:00 A.M. to 10:00 A.M.   105

Notebook: Resident-Care Conference   110

6. Bridges to the Community   114

Notebook: The New Admission   122

7. Separation and Adaptation: The Passage   124

Notebook: The Kitchen   141

Contents

Voice: Ida Kanter   149

8. The Limits of Exchange   153

Voice: Bernice Meyerhov   180

9. Liminality in the Nursing Home: The Endless Transition   183

Notebook: Resident-Care Conference   210

10. Summary and Conclusion   214

Voice: Priscilla Frails, Nursing Assistant   221

Notes   225

References   233

Index   241

Tables

1. Residents with dementia   43
2. Goldfarb mental status test   44
3. Characteristics of total institutions   98

What is time? A mystery, a figment—and all-powerful. . . . Now is not then, here not there, for between them lies motion. But the motion by which one measures time is circular, is in a closed circle; and might almost equally well be described as rest, as cessation of movement—for the there repeats itself constantly in the here, the past in the present.

Thomas Mann, *The Magic Mountain*

Nothing should be more expected than old age: nothing is more unforseen . . .

Simone de Beauvoir, *The Coming of Age*

Danger lies in transitional states. . . . the person who must pass from one to another is himself in danger and emanates danger to others. . . . he cannot help his abnormal situation.

Mary Douglas, *Purity and Danger*

Preface

The life cycle is truly a cycle, and I have been struck by this truth many times in the process of researching and writing this book. I came to the study of nursing-home residents out of the dawning understanding of my own aging. The first indelible experiences within my family, my early, deep love for my grandparents, and, finally, the creating by my husband and me of our own children came together into a wish to understand this cycle better.

Different ages both divide and unite us, and yet, throughout the cycle, one's sense of oneself remains constant. I wonder what will face me as an old person; I am concerned how nursing homes will be when I may need one. I have forced myself to confront this possibility even though old age seems so remote to the young who claim health and vigor as unexamined rights.

In analyzing one American nursing home in the early 1980s, I tried to understand what ingredients make for the "uneasy life" I found there. I consider three theoretical ideas. First, impersonal, organizational principles account for many of the conflicts and the divisiveness in the institution. Staff members are socialized within their professions to different worldviews, which act as barriers to effective teamwork. Hierarchies and territorialities of the bureaucratic structure lock staff members together in predictable battles. Second, nursing-home residents are placed in a mostly passive and receiving role: needy of care and services, they have little opportunity to make decisions or to help one another or the institution in which they live. Finally, and most significantly, the nursing-home residents find themselves without anchor in a rite of passage between adulthood and death. This rite of passage is gloomy because it is shorn of community support. The nursing-home existence is a long transition, seemingly endless and without goal. In this passage, residents experience a liminality without ritual and without communitas—that is, without the bonding and the support of others who help articulate the meaning of the passage. Nonetheless, glimmers of bonding in this nursing home arise out of the physical therapy setting, but these instances are all the more poignant because of their rarity in the total nursing-home experience.

The theoretical chapters are interwoven with my observations of events and transcribed tape recordings of individual people under the headings "Notebook" and "Voice." This material helps the reader imagine nursing-home life and judge my formulations. These sections are presented without comment to show experiences that contributed to forming my argument. They are subjective and personal, and while they are authentic, the observations are necessarily incomplete.

This study was undertaken with the help of many people to whom I remain indebted and connected. I owe thanks to the people who permitted me to do this work and to those who supported, guided, and taught me throughout the research and writing. I am indebted to the administrators and trustees of the (pseudonymous) Franklin Nursing Home, who generously permitted me complete access to the institution. Various members of the Harrison community who were involved with the nursing home also spent time with me, for which I am most grateful. Staff members within the home patiently explained and explored its ways with me and were generous with their time and expertise. Throughout my research I was impressed by the willingness to help that everyone at the home expressed and repeatedly demonstrated. I was also impressed by the goodwill of the staff members and the complexity and arduousness of their work. Most important, I am deeply grateful to the residents of the Franklin Nursing Home, who have taught me so much and have immeasurably enriched my life by allowing me to know them. I have changed everyone's names and some key traits to preserve privacy. In the interests of confidentiality, it is impossible to name those who have been so valuable to this research and to me personally. You know who you are, and I thank you.

Stanley M. Aronson, William O. Beeman, George L. Hicks, and Lucile F. Newman provided invaluable confrontation, stimulation, and help to me during the research and writing. Roger Sanjek enabled me to see new connections and helped me shape the work into its present form. I have been aided by the comments of several other readers of the manuscript in its various stages. I thank Kathleen Cushman, Marsha Fretwell, Valerie Gordon, Henry Izeman, Moses Kaufman, Rachel Kaufman, Seth Lieberman, Robert Nathan, Daniel Asa Rose, Josef Sternberg, and Hugo Taussig for their thoughtful readings and helpful feedback. My parents, Anne and Gilbert Rose, and my husband, Paul, provided me with honest and careful criticisms couched in a love that sustained me.

My indebtedness to all these people is in part complemented, I hope, by my independence from them. My thoughts have developed in contact with theirs over the years; we weave together some coherence that simultaneously delineates our separateness. The greatest source and resource remains the concentric circles of my family— my parents, brothers, sister, their spouses, their children, my husband's family, the memories of my grandparents, my aunts and uncles and cousins, my partnership with Paul, and the promise of continuity that is our children. In this regard, it is most lovely that our last baby, Lily Susanna, was born some hours after I finished this book, joining Sonja, Aaron, and David. Her birth completes this important cycle for Paul and me—and in so doing, begins a brand new one all over again.

RENÉE ROSE SHIELD

Seekonk, Massachusetts

Uneasy Endings

Notebook:
7:00 A.M. to 3:00 P.M.

6:50 A.M. *I arrive at the Franklin Nursing Home and say hello to the security guard at the front desk. He comments that it is a beautiful day.*
7:00. *I'm on the second floor. I had arranged to follow the charge nurse, Eileen, around today during her shift, but am told that she's in the hospital, sick. Aymara, the nurse from the pool, has been called in to replace Eileen. She grudgingly agrees to let me shadow her today.*

Jeanine, a nurse, is on the phone, calling Bernice, the supervisor, to get more staff to be on today. So far they're short. Hal, an orderly, is reading a sex magazine and laughing with Sayzie, a nurse with black curly hair. Hal says there aren't enough pictures. I hear a constant beeping sound, which no one answers. Some of the residents are walking around. Others in the dining area are sitting, reading. Jeanine is grumpy and says there are only seven people on today, which is not enough. She sips coffee from a cup decorated obscenely. The staff members milling around comment approvingly about the cup. Jeanine says she'll give one to Eileen to cheer her up.
7:15. *Nurses' report is in the dining room. We sit around a table near the door. I'm asked to tell what I'm doing there. I explain that I am an anthropologist and want to follow Aymara around for the entire shift. I'm interested in what it's like to live here. "What life?" asks Hal pointedly. They introduce themselves: in addition to Sayzie, Hal, and Aymara are three nursing assistants named Astrid, Georgia, and Lizzie and an orderly, Julio. Another nurse, Jessie, comes in, and finally one more nurse, Alma, joins us. When Hal asks me if I'm Jewish, I say yes. He complains that when someone went to the hospi-*

tal, Hal was asked to attend that person for the length of stay. Of course he didn't do it, but imagine the nerve of asking him to go to the hospital to feed the resident! Other people without family have no one to push for them, he adds.

Aymara starts the report and announces that I'll follow her around. The jokes about this make me feel a little uncomfortable. Included in the report is that Joel Kaplan has died and that Louis Goldberg is okay today. Lizzie is very sleepy, and Astrid kids her.

7:30.   Report is over. Aymara returns to the nurses' station and uses the phone. Several of the others stay in the dining room. The television has been on all along. Staff members are smoking. I'm told that if I want to smoke it would be all right. Aymara tells me it's a "heavy" floor; this means that there is much to do, and that's why they have to have more staff on. A resident, Charlie Kassin, is here now, checking on things. I ask him how Hannah Kleinberg, his cousin, is doing. He has come to the floor to find out. Aymara goes back into the dining room. She tells various staff people who should have his or her temperature taken, and she's trying to find out who needs to stay in bed today. Hal says that he's going home at noon today since he's on overtime. Jeanine reminds him that Bernice says if he's going to come in for overtime, he should stay the whole shift. Hal disagrees and says they're lucky he came in at all. A female employee is sullenly wiping the counter of the nurses' station. Aymara tells her about a spill someplace, and she answers, "I don't mop."

7:45.   Julio turns up the television in the dining room. We're all in there again as Aymara is still checking on what everyone's going to be doing during the shift. Paul McCartney is being interviewed on the Today show. Lizzie is excited and Astrid joins her closer to the set. Aymara finds out which nursing assistants and orderlies are assigned to which residents.

8:00.   Aymara says, "Don't anyone give me trouble today, okay?" Everyone answers her with an exaggerated "Of course not, Aymara." As a pool nurse, Aymara is called when someone is out sick. This is her favorite floor, but she can get assigned anywhere, depending on the need. She'll even fill in for LPNs at times, although she's an RN. She excuses herself to phone Bernice for the latest on who's coming in, and tells Bernice that Georgia still isn't in. Then she goes down the hall to answer the beeping signal, then back to the dining room to ask who is in charge of the resident whose beeper is on; now she determines who needs a laxative or an enema today. Seeing Ernie Schechter's light

[2]

on, she goes to his room and says, "Hal will get you up in a few minutes, honey. Okay, dear? It's eight in the morning. Okay, darling? He'll be down in a minute." Turning to me, she says that one has to baby them sometimes; they're old and need special attention.

8:15.   We're sitting in the little cubicle behind the nurses' station, having coffee. Everyone is smoking, except Aymara and me. Jeanine and Sayzie are talking about marriage. Jeanine recounts how their bed was fixed up by friends in the Portuguese tradition on their return from their honeymoon: hotdogs and perfume and other things were put into the bed. A resident comes over to the nurses' station and asks, "Who's giving me my bath?" He is told that Hal will give him his bath after lunch.

8:30.   We're still in the cubicle. Sidney Black, a resident, comes over, and Sayzie tells him to change his shirt because it has some stains on it. Aymara and Sayzie are filling out forms. Jeanine is at the nurses' station. Dolly, a private-duty nurse for Mrs. Herman, arrives. After a few minutes sitting, she says, "Well, I guess I ought to go give Madame Herman her bath." The phone rings: Bernice wants to have the time sheets brought to her office. Aymara and Jeanine ask each other where the time sheets are. Aymara tells me she likes to have all these things straightened out. The physical therapist, Jean, comes in. The phone rings again: where are the time sheets? The phone rings several more times. Aymara tells me that sometimes when she's at home she answers her phone automatically with "Second floor, Aymara." Eileen calls from the hospital. Jeanine talks to her; then Aymara calls her back to find out how she is and when she's coming back. Maybe next week.

8:45.   The supply man comes and tries to determine whether more oxygen tanks are needed. They keep winding up on other floors, such as the fourth floor, where they aren't needed as much. The tank used for Joel Kaplan needs to be replaced since he's died, and they have to be ready for the next person who needs oxygen. The supply man leaves and comes back a few times to report on where he has looked for the missing tank. Turns out it was on the fourth floor. Aymara goes back to filling out Blue Cross forms. She's checking others she has done to make sure that she did them correctly. Joel Kaplan was such a nice man, she tells me. The day before yesterday he had fallen asleep and then fell out of his chair. She had to give him oxygen.

9:00.   Aymara continues. She called Mr. Kaplan's family because she thought he might be near death. The family member kept pressing

Aymara to say exactly "what does that mean," and Aymara told the person that Mr. Kaplan might die and that she did not want his death to be too much of a shock. The family member was grateful. Sometimes the staff member who promises to call the family with news doesn't do it. Aymara says she always tries to call; it's only right.

Aymara talks to me now about favoritism among the nurses and why she thinks the other floors get better admissions than does the second floor. She fills out forms and tells me that a lot of time is spent doing this kind of thing. Others may say that nurses don't do anything when they are sitting at the nurses' station, but they always have a lot of paperwork to do. Now one of the nursing assistants tells Aymara that Ruby Kapstein has a bedsore.

9:15. As Jessie, an LPN, arrives, Aymara says they have too much help. Jessie says she'll do whatever they want—dressings, treatments—even though she's a nurse. But perhaps there won't be so much work today: Mrs. Carey and Mrs. Kleinberg are in the hospital now. Jessie asks, "How's Joel Kaplan?" When Aymara tells her that he died, Jessie exclaims, "Didn't I tell you? I knew it!" Then, to me: "You're happy when someone nice like that dies—without suffering from the cancer. It was good he had a bad heart. If you have a strong heart, it's bad. I've seen it." Then Jessie asks me, "Are you the anthropologist? I pictured someone with monkeys." I laugh and can't think of anything to say in answer. One of the nurses discusses a resident with gangrene. Sayzie, Jessie, and Aymara talk about how they prefer to be on a heavy floor where they can do "real" nursing. Other floors are boring because the medical-nursing needs of the residents are far less than here. Someone tells us that Eileen is coming out of the hospital on Saturday and that she'll be back to work then, too. There is amazement about this news. Aymara gets back to the Blue Cross forms.

9:30. Aymara and I go downstairs to bring the time sheets and the Blue Cross forms to Bernice. Aymara and Bernice talk about whether Eileen will be back Saturday or not. She had better not do as many double shifts as she was doing before, they say. It's not fair to the others who want overtime. Bernice notices that I'm carrying a book about Alzheimer's disease. If the book is about drugs, she's not interested, she says with a dismissing wave. She tries to keep up with some things, but the medication world has changed too fast and is too complex for her to stay current. Bernice says her sister called her this morning to tell her she read in the paper that Joel Kaplan died.

Bernice didn't even know. "What a brave man," she comments. "Dear God, let me be like that when I go."

Bernice asks me to leave so that they can talk privately. I go outside the office and wait. After a few minutes Aymara emerges, and we go back upstairs.

9:45. Jessie tells Aymara that the suprapubic tube on Charlie Rosenbaum is really bad. Together Jess, Aymara, and I go to his room to check. I wait outside the door, but am told later that I could have gone in. Aymara tells Jessie that they have to determine when the tube was last changed. Aymara goes to check Ernie Schechter, whose light at the nurses' station is on. He's on the toilet and wants her to tell him if he's moved his bowels or not. She says he has, and she tells him that she can't help him get up because of her back but that she'll get Hal to come and help lift him. We go back to the nurses' station. "Where's Hal?" Aymara asks and is told that he on a break. Aymara checks the files and finds that Mr. Rosenbaum's tube was changed a few weeks ago. It's time to change it. We go back to his room with Jessie, and I wait outside while the procedure is done. Mr. Rosenbaum's roommate, Mr. Abrams, asks for his bath. Aymara answers him, "Hal's coming, Mr. Abrams. Don't worry, darling. You've got to wait. You're not his only patient. He's on his break right now." I hear the Phil Donahue show on TV in the room.

10:00. We go back to the nurses' station again. Aymara notes the procedure in the chart. A tiny woman looking like a fragile bird and dressed in a too-large but springlike yellow suit walks tentatively by the nurses' station, gingerly touching the counter as she goes. We introduce ourselves. I compliment her on her dress, and she seems very pleased. Dolly, the private duty nurse, sees her and says, "Hi, little peach," and hugs her. The woman's name is Millie Siskind. A male resident who passes Millie kisses her cheek while we all look on. Dolly says to me, "Isn't that cute? Look at that. Poor little things."

Aymara is putting slips of paper in the charts. Julio can't figure out whether Jerry Albert had the enema or not. It wasn't written in the chart, but Mr. Albert said he did have the enema. Aymara tells Julio to check other records to track it down. Julio comes back and reports that Frank gave Jerry Albert the enema but didn't write it down in the chart.

10:15. Aymara tells Hal to get Ernie Schechter off the toilet. Millie Siskind walks carefully back and forth by the nurses' station. Sayzie puts her hands on Millie's cheeks and then hugs her. Sayzie says to

[5]

me, "She's so sweet—doesn't bother anyone." Jeanine tells Aymara that Murray Hachen needs a Foley catheter. Aymara continues to enter things in the various charts. She tells Julio to give Mr. Abrams his shower now. Julio says he will do it later, but Aymara says he will have another shower to do then. Julio insists that he knows how long it takes to do the shower, and he'll do it later. Aymara tells him that to do "quality care," he should not rush and do it now, but Julio still claims that he can do the two showers in a half hour. A resident, Mr. Sager, walks past the nurses' station. He's reading a book about Herzl, which, when I ask about it, he says is quite "dry." He tells a staff person that he is writing a book, as well. There is some mild interest.

10:30. Someone from the activities department is here. She asks me, "What kind of an anthropologist are you, anyhow?" I start to explain, but when I see that Aymara has gone I have to follow her. Aymara and Sayzie are putting a catheter on Mr. Hachen. I ask to watch. Sure. Murray Hachen lies on his back looking at the ceiling. I feel that I should introduce myself and ask his permission to be there, but he seems to be trying to make himself invisible during the procedure, so I decide to say nothing. Sayzie holds his penis and tells him what she is doing. Aymara is on the other side of the bed, watching and listening. Hal stands quietly and stoically, as if at attention. I'm next to Sayzie, near Mr. Hachen's feet. Sayzie explains that this is easier on a man than on a woman. She inserts the catheter. At first there is no urine, but then it comes. They all comment on how much there is. Sayzie inspects the urine and comments that it's cloudy and needs to be analyzed.

Back in the cubicle behind the nurses' station, everyone talks about diets. A nurse from another floor brags about her crazy diet and demonstrates her fabulous slimmed-down body.

10:45. Aymara resumes charting. Sayzie comments that Mr. Abrams is a selfish man. "Then again, what do I know?" she asks: apparently he was in the Holocaust. Still, he only thinks about himself, and has numerous requests of the staff all day. She's reached the point where she almost never hears him anymore, just like with her children when they were little. Does Aymara know that Mr. Feinberg has cancer of the bladder? asks Sayzie. Yes, answers Aymara absently.

11:00. Aymara goes downstairs. She tells me that she'd rather go by herself and she'll only be a minute. A staff person can't find the treatment-room keys. Aymara comes back and resumes charting. I am uncomfortable that Aymara acts like she does not want me shadowing her.

11:15. I hear someone yelling. Apparently it is Ruby Kapstein, the same person whose bedsore was reported earlier in the morning. Jeanine says, "My headache is killing me."

11:30. Aymara says she's going to lunch now. She makes it clear to me that she's going "out" and has errands to do. I decide to observe the residents' lunch, which has just begun in the dining room. I sit along the glass wall. One of the residents waves to me. I wave back. A woman is being fed by the nurse Alma. The woman scrunches up her face and repeatedly asks, "Am I all right?" Alma says, "You should say, 'I am all right!' In a tearful voice the woman repeats, "I am all right," and then, "Am I all right?" several times, and then weeps. Alma reassures her, stroking her shoulders and her hair, patiently repeating to her that she is all right and that everything is fine. The resident says she can't swallow the food in her mouth. Alma gets it out for her. After a few minutes, the woman asks again, anxiously, "Am I all right?" and Alma responds reassuringly again. Her crying comes and goes. I have seen her many times before. Her face seems set in a frozen scowl, and because she has frightened me, I've always avoided her. This time I'm determined to let her eyes meet mine. They do. After a minute, she smiles. I smile back.

11:45. Julio gets Mr. Kravits set up for lunch. He's asleep in a wheelchair a few seats down from me against the glass wall. Julio gently wakens him, tells him what is happening, that it is Thursday, that it is lunch time, and he puts his tray in front of him and places a bib around his chest. He threads the ties beneath the frozen arms and between his shoulders and stiffened neck. Julio explains to me that Mr. Kravitz is 96 years old.

12:00 P.M. Jeanine tells me that she's feeling sicker. People are finishing their lunches. Mr. Sager says it was a good meal and hurries out. Julio asks him to slow down so as not to hurt himself. Astrid asks me to have lunch with a few of them in several minutes.

12:15. I go to lunch with Alma, Gert, a fourth-floor nurse, Georgia, and Julio. We talk about Julio's new baby. There are labor and delivery stories and accounts of what it's like to have a newborn around. We commiserate about sleepless nights. A woman I have seen on the various floors getting drinks and little things for people tries to join us. She speaks with difficulty and seems deaf. Alma invites her to sit with us, but there isn't room, so she moves to another table. Alma is concerned that her feelings were hurt.

1:15. Back upstairs. Aymara is charting again. Everyone is being readied for the monthly birthday party held at 2:00 downstairs. One

[7]

of the wandering residents, Mr. Black, has gone out a door, setting off the alarm. Hal is sent to get him, but it takes a while to locate him and bring him back. Astrid passes a resident. "Oh, Mr. Schwartz," she remarks kindly, "You've stained your shirt at lunch. Go on down to your room, and I'll be there in a moment to help you put on a new one. Wait for me." He looks down at his shirt, nods slowly, and proceeds down the hallway to his room.

1:30. *Aymara is in the little cubicle talking with Bernice. Some of the others are there as well. I feel that I shouldn't join them because they seem to be complaining.*

1:45. *I decide to join them in the cubicle. Aymara motions to me: would I please leave since this conversation is private. I leave. More residents are wheeled into the elevator to go downstairs for the party. They are dressed up, and the women wear corsages.*

2:00. *Aymara comes out and tells me it's okay for me to come in. They had been talking about a problem with an LPN and the union, and it's straightened out now. Astrid wants to know what I've been writing in my orange notebook. I tell her that I've taken notes on what I've noticed during the shift. Everyone talks about dieting. Almost everyone goes into the nurses' station now. Jessie takes out the sex magazine that Hal had been reading at 7:00 A.M. As she walks down the hall, Hal goes after her. The snack tray comes up and Julio gives the residents tea, juice, and cookies. Aymara calls a doctor on the phone about one of the residents who has a cough. She questions why the resident is on codeine. Bernice tells me that sometimes doctors don't prescribe the right things.*

2:15. *Ruby Kapstein's bedsore is on her foot. Harriet, a social worker, comes to the nurses' station and tells Aymara that it "would have been really nice if Sarah had gone to the birthday party. She wanted to go, but didn't know that she could go." Aymara gasps apologetically and tells Harriet that she completely forgot. After Harriet leaves, Aymara resumes charting. Hal is still looking for Mr. Black. Julio asks Sayzie if she's doing a double shift today. "Are you kidding?" she exclaims, and he giggles. He's not doing one either. He works weekends and Thursdays. The rest of the time he is in school studying to be a nurse. He wishes he were allowed to do more procedures here, but because he hasn't technically completed his degree yet, he is not permitted. However, at the hospital he would be allowed to do more, and he resents the restrictions here.*

Mr. Black is back. Julio takes him upstairs to the eye clinic. Aymara is charting and says it has been a typical day. She likes being busy, but there's much paperwork, especially if a doctor has been in to see a resident. Several nursing assistants and orderlies are in the dining room near the television set, joking loudly. Lizzie is acting out a story. 2:30. Alma sighs, "It's almost the end of the day." She says that residents can feel when the shift is about to end. They get somewhat anxious, and want to know who will be on, who will have them. "They have an inner clock." Sayzie tells Aymara that no one's from the pool except Gloria, the nursing assistant. Aymara is writing the nurses' reports about each of the residents to be read at the beginning of the next shift. Someone takes the cloudy urine from Murray Hachen to the lab.

2:45. The 3:00–11:00 shift starts trickling in. A big jovial man, an orderly, dances into the nurses' station. I meet Sandy, the charge nurse for the next shift, who does not smile though she agrees to my being on her shift sometime. Everybody hangs around the nurses' station. Someone starts to punch out but is stopped because there is a rule that they can't leave until replacements have come, and not enough people have arrived for the next shift.

Alma tells Jeanine that she has a good Catholic joke for her. They lean against the railing of the nurses' station: A boy is bounced from school to school, never doing well. Finally, his parents enroll him in a Catholic school, and when the first report card comes, lo and behold, he's gotten all A's. So his parents ask him why he is doing so well. The boy answers, "Well, I saw that they took a kid and nailed him up on the wall, so I knew they meant business!" Jeanine pulls back in disgust and horror. "Alma," she says intently, "That's blasphemy. That's blasphemy. How can you tell such a joke?" Alma is surprised that Jeanine doesn't enjoy the joke.

It's almost 3:00. Everyone punches the time clock. I thank Aymara for letting me accompany her. She says it was fine with her, and I'm welcome to do it again. I catch the elevator with most of the nursing assistants and orderlies in it. Downstairs, the birthday party is in full swing. A band is playing, and the entire hall is filled with residents, staff, family members. I look carefully at the residents, and they appear to be enjoying the music, which is saxophoney and schmaltzy. Time for me to go.

[9]

[1]

Anthropology in an
American Nursing Home

Standing apart on a side street, a handsome, modern building houses old people confined by frailty. On nice days some of them sit in chairs by the entrance and chat. Some stare ahead; some of them walk carefully, tentatively picking their way with walkers, or attended by nursing assistants or family companions. Flowers and pachysandra are planted attractively nearby. The Franklin Nursing Home is the long-term care facility where over two hundred people live, most of them in their eighties or nineties.[1] They are unable to care for themselves on their own, and they live in the nursing home for an average of four years, time enough to call it home. They are cared for, nourished, protected, kept from harm and, until the end, from death. Almost all of them are Jewish; most immigrated from Eastern Europe or Russia at the beginning of the century. Many have no family to care for them.

This book is an anthropological study of the Franklin Nursing Home, located in Harrison, an industrial city in the northeastern United States. It is a special nursing home in many ways. It is a nonprofit, Jewish nursing home which, because it receives federal funds, is open to all. It is a "good" nursing home, with high staffing ratios and better facilities and services than most nursing homes. It enjoys important ties with the Jewish community, which are crucial to its financial survival. Many of the residents knew each other before admission, and many Jewish holidays are celebrated here.

Why Anthropology?

In this book I attempt to discover the mundane, ordinary life of this nursing home. When I began my study I had certain assumptions and expectations I wanted to test. Interested in the ongoing dailiness of the residents' lives, I learned at the outset that the meaning of nursing home life is better revealed in small, repetitive details of routine life than in dramatic events. Though part of me wanted to simplify reality by attempting an exposé full of startling discoveries pulled from undercover espionage, I also expected to discover a community of concerned and caring individuals striving together to ease the passage of the frail elderly during their last years. Though it might have been cathartic to assign blame or exonerate victims, life in the nursing home is too complicated for exaggerated portrayals. Instead, a complex tangle of good intentions, budgetary constraints, federal and state regulations, bureaucratic officiousness, professional dictates, union loyalties, family divisiveness, religious prescriptions, human frailty, humane desires, and idiosyncratic individuality of a particularly American type seem to me to characterize life in this nursing home.

Perhaps the most basic endeavor that anthropologists perform is that of untangling what the members of a society say they do from what their behaviors indicate they actually do. The tendency of people everywhere to idealize behavior is complicated by myths that people entertain about themselves and about those in other cultures. Sometimes the opposite of idealization occurs instead. Denigration—of one's own culture or that of others—also arises from confusing the real with the ideal. For example, Americans often assume that their treatment of the elderly is shameful. Though most American elderly live close to their children and are institutionalized only after all other alternatives have been tried (Shanas 1979, Mace and Rabins 1981, Brody 1977), the folk notion that Americans dump their elderly relatives in substandard nursing homes persists, and the belief that being old in America is in sharp and disgraceful contrast to being old in traditional, non-Western cultures lingers despite continual refutation (Nydegger 1983).

Cultural anthropologists study human beings and their cultural institutions. We are interested in humans as they live today in all parts of the world, and to understand the variety of human behavior, we utilize comparison. Anthropologists who study non-Western cultures bring to bear the understanding that what they observe is both different from and similar to other cultures, including their own. Increasingly, American cultural anthropologists have come home to study their own cultures. This development is doubly important. It fulfills the original enterprise of anthropology: to study others in order to better understand ourselves. Second, we cannot assume a knowledge of Americans without investigating them with the same methods and questions that we use for others. Because people in the United States come from many kinds of cultures, the variety cannot be understood intuitively. What Americans share is not immediately ascertainable. Anthropological investigation reveals patterns and distinctions that can help us understand who we are.

Whenever we study anything human, our biases are with us. Though we strive to be neutral, objectivity remains an unattainable goal. It is a truism in anthropology that the observer changes what he or she observes. Trying to be both in and out of the culture through participant observation, the anthropologist finds that the boundaries of who "they" are, who "we" are, what constitutes the interaction between us, and how it varies according to the situation are murky and indistinct.

Many academic disciplines assume that aging itself is a problem. Anthropology questions the problem-oriented approach because it has impeded our ability to learn who the elderly are, what they think, how they organize their experiences, and how they are varied. Doing anthropology in an American nursing home made me focus on several questions. What is it like to live in a nursing home? How do people make the decision (or have the decision made for them) to enter a nursing home? What are the people concerned about? What are their days like? What does it feel like to be old? What do the old people have in common with each other? How are they old? How are they like me? What is age and why is it important?

These are difficult questions precisely because at first glance they seem simple and obvious, intuitively clear. We answer them automatically by our tacit assumptions, and these assumptions are idiosyncratically personal as well as cultural. Our assumptions are neat encapsulations of what is firmly entrenched in our minds as natural; but because they are assumptions that we usually do not reflect upon, we do not realize that they may not be shared. And if they are not shared, they cannot be natural in the same way that biological structures are natural. Anthropologists like to say that we make the familiar strange and we make the strange familiar. In the process we learn how we are different from and similar to others.

[12]

Making the Familiar Strange

Making the familiar strange is the reverse of what those anthropologists who work in cultures not their own do. When an anthropologist leaves the familiarity of his or her own society to venture into one that is explicitly and immediately different, the task is to decipher the initially incomprehensible ways of the culture and render them meaningful in the anthropologist's terms. In some ways the anthropologist who goes to another culture has an advantage because the differences between his own society and the one he studies are prominent. Similarities are less apparent and emerge later. The anthropologist Robert Murphy, in investigating his own culture of quadriplegia, has commented on the undeserved objectivity that foreign fieldwork seems to command:

> There was a time when anthropology rested its claim for "objectivity" on its concern with other, often exotic, cultures. Since we did not share the values and biases of our subjects, it was argued, we saw them with a clear, nonpartisan eye. This was self-serving nonsense, for the truth is that our perceptions in ethnographic research are deeply affected by our personalities, by the language categories into which we sort our reality, by our education, by all the overburden of our own culture. And, as we get deeper into our research, the people's own interpretation of their culture provides an added coloration of our views, a further skewing of our perceptions. Our need to reduce all our data to a tidy system is just as much an attempt to cope with the sensory chaos of a world we do not fully understand as an exercise in science. And it is subject to the same errors and uncertainties. (1987:176)

An anthropologist studying his own society deliberately places himself outside the ways of the culture in a self-conscious way. He questions what he already thinks he knows. The purpose is thus to see the arbitrariness of what ordinarily looks normal and routine. Agar has commented on the difficulty of this kind of fieldwork: "You might think that doing ethnography in one's own society would be less stressful. I find it more so. . . . In ethnography of the traditional sort, there is a period of travel and adjustment of the field setting, followed by a long period of time in residence. After the fieldwork is over, one travels home and readjusts to the home culture. When you work in your own society, you cross the line between the field and home often and rapidly" (1980:52).

Making the familiar strange is both an uncomfortable and an excit-

[13]

ing process. We are eased by routines and assumptions. Questioning them disrupts the illusion we usually protect: that there is coherence and order to how we go about our lives. If we question the links between events, then we have to rethink how to make those connections. When we try to untangle the familiar, to question why we believe what we do is obvious, we can learn about the values that make up our rationale for behaving as we do. When we uncover some of these values, we arrive at the convictions that motivate us, and we can begin to understand, and perhaps even reconcile, differences between us. For example, many of the things that nurses in the nursing home do are motivated by their adherence to a principle to maintain life. Many social workers in the nursing home, on the other hand, question that assumption and are motivated by principles having to do with maintaining a good quality of life. Some of the nurses and social workers spoke about the underlying conflict in these terms. The nurses and the social workers frequently come into conflict when their work so intimately involves the frail elderly. Articulating the assumptions that underlie the different behaviors helps us understand why the behaviors are different.

Trying to make the familiar strange in this nursing home was eerie for me. I was investigating my own culture, and many of the residents reminded me of my grandparents and European relatives. It was a comfortable setting in some ways. Though I do not speak Yiddish, I could converse easily with them in English, and I was familiar with various Yiddish phrases. I had heard stories and expressions similar to theirs in my upbringing. In order to understand their specific experiences, however, I had to pluck myself out of this comfortable stance. They knew that I was studying the nursing home, not merely chatting amiably. I had to question what I heard and not let their stories and observations pile up in the familiarly convenient category I already knew from my childhood.

Listening was a task charged with difficulty and capable of providing new meaning. I had to prevent myself from being lulled by familiar linguistic phrases and stories of pogroms and passage. I had to hear each person anew, and I had to obstruct my easy interpretations of what I did hear. I attempted to listen openly, freshly. I asked what I thought they would think were stupid questions. Their answers taught me new things. My familiarity gave me a seemingly easy access to the reminiscences and present concerns of these people, but this familiarity had to be combated constantly, as well.

[14]

The openness of this kind of listening is uniquely anthropological. We bring ourselves to the field situation and utilize our biases, hunches, assumptions, and other facets of our personalities and intelligence, but we hold them at bay at the same time. We suspend expectation. If the prejudging is not held at arm's length, the listening is tainted and the learning is stunted. When I asked the question, "What is it like to live in a nursing home?" I did not know the answer, not having lived in a nursing home. Thus, I treated the temptingly familiar and predictable as traps to be sniffed at warily and examined with extra scrutiny.

Making the Strange Familiar

On the other hand, feeling at first familiar with these old people and their culture did not negate what was strange and alien to me about them and their setting. The net effect was that I never felt comfortable either going by my assumptions or avoiding what seemed distasteful.

The sensory experience was immediately strange to me, but over time I became acclimated to it. Though the Franklin Nursing Home is clean, smells of urine were always unpleasant and surprising to encounter. There were disturbing sounds: people moaning from down the hall, people crying out, one old person scolding another harshly, the sounds of weeping and of protest. Sights too were jarring and sometimes threatening. The first time I walked into the large sitting room, which was in use as the cafeteria, I was startled to see people staring at me. Some looked inquisitive, some looked baffled and uncomprehending, some looked as though I had disturbed their equanimity by being there. I was initially frightened by their appearance: one hunched far over in his chair, eyes bulging, thin hair splayed; another being spoon-fed; another staring ahead, unreacting. When I smiled and said hello to certain individuals, their faces became animated. I tried it out on those whose faces held mine in an unrelenting stare. My smile sometimes, though not always, activated a smile in response. This reassuring human contact helped alleviate my initial alarm.

Some things that made me uncomfortable were more cognitive and emotional than sensory. Though some staff members spoke to the residents as if they were adults, and others spoke with much warmth and tenderness, others spoke in ways that bothered me. The residents were often rebuked, patronized, and infantilized. I believe the assumption that underlies this stance is that old people are not like us. Staff members often coached me with generalizations about how old people are. Behaviors that I asked about were often explained in terms such as "that's the way they are when they're old." Though residents were often treated as individuals, there was a tendency to regard them as a category and as other than "us." Baffling behaviors were explained as due to old age rather than to individual factors.

Some staff members seemed to believe that the old people were as different as another species. Looking back, I believe I initially shared this assumption of difference. Increasingly, however, I was jarred away from accepting this gap. Instead, I came to understand that what others and I thought of as different and discontinuous was in fact shared and continuous. The strange was becoming familiar. In the beginning I felt inalienably young encountering people who were inalienably old. As I came to know many of the old people, I recognized more things we had in common—more young things about them, more old things about me, more links between us than gaps separating us. I found this continuity disturbing. I recognized that the perceived gap between old and young creates an illusion for the young that inhibits understanding their potentiality as old. Understanding that the separation was artificial made me recognize that the old people were more familiar than I had thought, or than I wanted them to be, and this familiarity, too, was strange. When I began to imagine myself old, when I imagined living in a nursing home relying on others, when, in short, I began to identify with them and their existence, I realized that this book was about me. If we continue, we grow old, and this is how it could be for us. Making the strange familiar was disconcerting and alarming—too close for comfort—but a necessary realization.

This Anthropologist

The work of anthropology is interactive—the anthropologist listens to, speaks to, is corrected by, reacts to, learns from, gives to, and observes those he or she studies. For this reason I must describe myself. To describe only the object of study would distort the anthropological enterprise.

When I started fieldwork, my husband and I had three children,

[16]

aged 6, 4, and 1. Before I was a parent, I felt immune to the aging process. Once I had a child, however, I felt I participated in the life cycle and was aging.

While I had much in common with the old people I studied, particularly the women, there were vast differences between them and me. I was a mother with small children, and I was still going to school. When I would have to rush away from the nursing home to pick a child up at nursery school, the residents were glad that I conformed to a role they thought I should have. We talked about husbands and children easily, but with different orientations. I was mired in details of daily life, trying to balance disparate parts of my life and schedule with those of my family. I was juggling babysitters, teaching, visiting the nursing home, helping at the children's schools, cooking my family's meals. They, on the other hand, were understimulated, waiting for visits, killing time with recreational activities, counting minutes until lunch or the favorite soap opera. Their talk of husbands and children derived from memories, not from the immediacy of the present. I felt drained from the minutiae of the dailiness; they seemed starved for it. We had many experiences in common, but their vague, dreamlike memories contrasted with the pressures that were constant for me. When we talked about children, many of the women said that their child-rearing years had occupied such a short part of their lives from their present perspective that they could hardly be sure those years had been real. It was hard for me to believe this because my life was completely caught up in unending, repetitive days of child rearing that seemed as if they would continue forever.

My relationships with the employees and staff varied. When the social workers took me under their wings, I sought out nurses, nursing assistants, and orderlies so that they understood that I wanted to know about them too. Everyone tolerated me generously: though at times I felt that I was in the way, or I was accused of being a spy, more often it seemed that they wanted to air their grievances and tell stories about themselves and others. I, on the other hand, envied the staff members because each had certain defined jobs to do every day. I had to decide each day what questions to ask, to whom I should speak, where I was confused, needed information, and so forth. Though the exciting challenge of anthropology is to question what others take for granted, I often wished I could be like them and not question.

My interests about age, aging, time, continuity, old, young, childhood, old age, and so on were personal and pressing and at the same

[17]

time had theoretical and intellectual appeal. When I became a mother and made my parents into grandparents, they were reluctantly thrust into a new societal definition. Their friends began calling them "grandma" and "grandpa," and they did not like it. I wondered if they were now truly old. I felt a new link and continuity between my mother and me; she had really once been my age, frustrated, delighted, and sleep-deprived after I was born! On what is this continuity spanning many years based? How does it transcend or deny the linear way we usually think of time and age?

I had many wonderful memories of my own grandparents. My mother's parents had died when I was only 7, but I recalled their European smells and ways and warmth with particular vividness. My father's parents survived into their late seventies, and so I was privileged to know them from my childhood into my adulthood, and my perceptions and understandings of them changed gradually. I had known no one who had ever lived in a nursing home. Like many other Americans, nursing-home existence seemed to me to be a cruel fate for a long life. I wanted to know more about it.

I was particularly interested in rites of passage throughout the life cycle. Influenced by the work of the late Victor Turner and Barbara Myerhoff and by the classic studies of Claude Lévi-Strauss, Marcel Mauss, and Arnold van Gennep, I wanted to understand how transition points along the life span, particularly in the passage between middle age and old age, expose and perhaps resolve individual crises of change in culturally visible ways. Were there rituals that marked the entrance into the nursing home? Did they make old age and preparation for death easier? Were the residents in the nursing home bound by a shared fate and a common participation in these rituals?

Fieldwork: Expectations and Surprises

I selected the Franklin Nursing Home for study for several reasons. First of all, good nursing homes are not often studied. The fact that it is nonprofit and mostly Jewish made the likelihood of ritual richness and community feeling a high one. Most of the aged who are admitted there die there, and this is not the case for many nursing homes where temporary stays are common. The shared fate of the residents might also contribute to the formation of community within the nursing home, I reasoned. Further, the large size of the nursing home and the fact that individuals with varying physical and mental deficits reside there should result in complex heterogeneity. Finally, the affiliation of the nursing home with a neighboring university and medical school influenced the administrators to allow this research to be undertaken.

During the fourteen months of fieldwork, I went to the nursing home for several hours at a time at various times of day or night as frequently as I could. I observed and participated in whatever was going on. I often attended the weekly staff meetings held to assess individual residents. I spent time with groups of residents or with individual residents, talking and listening. I attended meals and activities, and I visited with residents in their rooms and at parties. Some of the residents allowed me to tape record their life histories. Everyone was eager to talk. It became apparent that not only were the residents anxious to have me visit and learn about them but the staff members wanted me to know what their roles and experiences were as well. When I introduced myself to the janitor, for example, he said impatiently, "I was wondering when you'd get around to me." This eagerness to talk was intensified because of a strike that was threatened in the first half of my fieldwork.

I watched a lot, as well. Participant observation involves the ability to stand by and be passive. Watching, writing notes on observations, wondering to myself what I was doing there, waiting for something to happen and not knowing what that something was supposed to be constitute a considerable proportion of fieldwork—an inchoate, unstructured endurance of viewing but not being a part of the doing. It is important to be ignored for periods of time in fieldwork, and it is necessary not to ask questions at times. This stance, which is often undesired but imposed upon us, enables us to see people behave. In watching behavior we are able to compare what people do with what they say they do. This attitude, which underlies what constitutes data, puts a necessary layer of complexity on findings that are obtained from survey research, questionnaires, and other similar tools that allow the subjects of investigation to restrict verbally what their researchers learn about them.

Many of the assumptions I had about the Franklin Nursing Home were not borne out by my study. I expected to find community feeling in the nursing home, first of all. Because most of the residents were Jewish and many of them knew each other before admission, I assumed there would be camaraderie, factions, fights, and much talking, joking, and arguing. Instead, I found little such community feeling.

There was sparse talk at mealtimes. I also expected that more would be shared by the residents. They had each had to leave homes to enter the nursing home; they each knew this was the last residence. Wouldn't this shared experience bind them together? Wouldn't Jewish custom and ritual and the fact that many of them came from Eastern Europe and Russia enhance their last years with shared traditions and heightened meaningfulness of Jewish ritual and belief? I found that not much was shared. The differences between them seemed to mean more to them. Holidays and rituals seemed thin, minimally performed. There was difficulty finding enough men to participate in early morning services. I had assumed that religion and tradition would become more important at the end of life, but this assumption was not borne out. I expected more involvement from Harrison community members than there seemed to be. I expected that the old people would be treated with respect in keeping with Jewish tradition, but I witnessed infantilization and nonperson treatment instead.

I was surprised that my expectations were not met. This book is about how my expectations were wrong.

Theoretical Context

The three main theoretical arguments I make in this book have been utilized separately by anthropologists to explain aspects of existence for the elderly. I believe that the three theories explain more when used together. My argument stems from Erving Goffman's description of total institutions, from reciprocity theory, and from rites-of-passage theory.

Goffman's (1961) *Asylums* is a vivid depiction of incarcerating institutions, which he termed "total" institutions, such as prisons, mental hospitals, boot camps, and nursing homes. Though he concentrated primarily on the mental hospital as the prototype, he maintained that the similarities between total institutions are more important than their differences. The key characteristics of total institutions are the definitive split between staff members and their charges or inmates, the rigid separation of the institution from the outside community, the imposition of the same routine for all inmates, and the fact that the daily activities of life, such as sleeping, working, and playing, are carried out under the same roof. The Franklin Nursing Home conforms in some ways to Goffman's description; how it does not conform needs to be explained in other terms. The utilization of the Goffman model, then, grounds my argument that other forces are at work in the nursing home.

Reciprocity theory describes how the ability to give and receive is related to power, choice, control, and definition as an adult. Glascock and Feinman (1981) have noted that nonindustrial societies usually distinguish the "intact aged" from the "decrepit aged." The distinction is often based on whether the individual is contributing in some way to the group or whether the group must support the individual. In many cases "death-hastening behaviors" are applied to those considered decrepit. The basic question is how do old people, removed from most mechanisms of exchange, maintain their relationships with others? There is little that the residents in the Franklin Nursing Home can use to exert control on others or on their situation. I argue that because nursing-home residents must receive, their ability to control their environment and themselves is crippled. Nonetheless, despite the curtailment of reciprocity, the residents manage to determine some aspects of their lives, often in ingenious and innovative ways.

Traditional anthropological theories of kinship systems and age-grading procedures in various cultures apply to the study of age and the elderly. Though much of the rites-of-passage literature illustrates how individuals are grouped by the society and pass from one status or age grade to the next in orderly succession, the literature also indicates the difficulty of the transitions. The reallocation of power within the society that is often the point of the rites-of-passage event causes strain and conflict among members (Gulliver 1963, Foner and Kertzer 1978).

In 1908 Arnold van Gennep's seminal *Les rites de passages* showed how rites of passage throughout the world have three parts: separation from the old status, transition between the old role and the new role (usually called *liminality*), and reincorporation into the new role. During rites of passage the initiate is receptive to learning about the new role into which he or she is about to be socialized. The stages are made routine and less stressful by the rituals that surround them. The liminal part of rites of passage is considered the most dangerous of the three segments. It is the time when a person is in neither one role nor another. Victor Turner (1967) developed the idea of liminality, expanding the concept to refer to all kinds of people and situations that are defined as neither in one category of social identity nor in another.

[21]

He stressed the positive aspects of liminality and used the term *communitas* to describe the togetherness the initiates in a rite of passage often share with one another.

I argue here that the aged individuals residing in the nursing home are undergoing a rite of passage: they are occupying the borderline, threshold state of the transition phase. They have been separated from their statuses as viable adults in the community, and not having died, they remain in the transition. Their liminality, however, is not marked by communitas. The Jewish community behaves ambivalently toward the nursing home: though supporting it financially, members of the community tend to avoid personal contact with residents. Most community rabbis refrain from involvement in the nursing home. Most physicians, not comfortable with the chronic and irreversible ailments of old age, tend to avoid the institution. In transition between adulthood and death, the nursing-home resident is perceived as "other"—neither adult nor dead. The ambivalent ways in which the residents are treated by both the community and the staff members within the nursing home indicate that the residents are perceived as dangerous, that they need to be avoided—as if they embody some of the death state they anticipate. But here another paradox surfaces: instead of enabling the resident to prepare for death, the nursing-home setting shushes the entire subject of death. Social and emotional withdrawal from the residents is coupled with vigorous physical interventions that maintain life. Thus the nursing home existence has an unreal, timeless quality to it. The passage has been interrupted and is little marked by sharing or ritual embellishments.

I argue that the dependency incurred from undergoing a ritual-less rite of passage and the dependency resulting from the reduced ability to exchange produce a more insidious dependency than would result from either form separately.

The belief that old people are like children was repeated often by the staff, and it intuitively struck me as wrong. Children as well as frail old people are seen as receivers who are little able to contribute. They are both deemed incapable of genuine help to the household or the economy or the nursing home, as the case may be. Labeling children and old people as incapable of contributing means that they are not worthy of full human status. Only adults who give and receive, who contribute, who participate in reciprocal relations with one another and in the larger society in which they live can be called adult with the connotations of full humanhood and responsible autonomy that American society designates. When old people and children are equated because of their perceived inability to contribute to the larger good, their status is demeaned, they are seen as demanding and selfish, and their dependencies are magnified.

In investigating the belief that old people are like children, I did not know whether my repugnance to this conviction was based on my romantic ignorance or whether there was validity to the belief. The literature was not helpful. Though writers have noted the existence of the belief, they have offered no convincing explanations. Utilizing reciprocity and rites-of-passage theory in conjunction with each other provides, I believe, a powerful tool for understanding the lives of nursing-home residents and explaining the existence of the belief that old people are like children. Bureaucratic rules in the nursing home and staff and community avoidance mechanisms toward the nursing-home residents are responses to the perceived danger of the liminal status of the residents. Liminality, together with restrictions on reciprocity, deepens the dependency and isolation of the residents. This process is synergistic, confounding, and spiraling.

As I have indicated, I am not interested in adding to the literature of the abominable nursing home. As Retsinas (1986) has eloquently argued, we tend too often to view the nursing home as corrupt and demeaning, and this predilection unfairly biases our seeing how nursing homes actually operate. Nursing homes are necessary for a certain percentage of our elderly population, and they will continue to be necessary. My purpose in this book is to argue that several underlying factors in the nursing home together create the difficult life of nursing-home residents. I have identified cultural and structural ingredients that I believe may be common and important in nursing homes in this country.

I am also taking the lead from others who have suggested that entrance into old age in the United States is a rite of passage for which there are few rituals: "Old people in industrial societies are, however, stranded in the liminal: exit signs are clearly marked, but reincorporation is not on the map" (Keith 1982a:82). Legesse (1979) agrees that there are no "obvious rites of transition" to mark these changes in our society though he doubts that in other societies the transitions are always as dramatic and sudden as heretofore described. Myerhoff notes the need for more work on rituals from the individual perspective: "The failure of anthropology to deal with the experiences of ritual participants—private, subjective, psychological, conscious, and un-

[23]

conscious—is an enormous barrier to our understanding of the subject" (1982:118).

The Turnerian bias for viewing the liminal state as a positive, creative, and bonding time for the initiates is rarely questioned. The nursing-home setting, however, may well be an instance of liminality without rituals and therefore without communitas. Though initiates undergoing liminality are often considered dangerous because of their marginality, the presence of rituals usually alleviates the tension. Without the rituals to explain and cushion the changes, however, avoidance of the initiates may substitute. If old people are liminal, this state may help explain why younger people often are unable to imagine themselves as potentially old (de Beauvoir 1972). Instead, the old seem exotic and alien. As Keith says, "The remarkable psychological feat is that so many of us are able to *maintain* a sense of distance from old people. . . . But instead of observing their explorations with self-interested curiosity, we transfer the exotic nature of the new social territory to the individuals exploring it, and keep our distance" (Keith 1982a:2).

In recent anthropological and sociological ethnographies of nursing homes, the community (or institution) is considered self-contained and cut off from the outside world, usually left undefined. Because links between the institution and the neighboring environment must be specified, I have tried to show the connections and the separations between the Franklin Nursing Home and the city in which it is located. I hope that the reader will penetrate beyond the stereotypes of the nursing home to see some of the complex dailiness of one quite good nursing home in the United States. Individual and group dramas are played out here as people struggle to achieve their needs, as they sit back and watch the passing scene, as staff members attend to the conflicting demands of their work and their clients, and as the inexorable routine of the institution maintains its steady pace.

Voice: Stanley Fierstein

Well, to begin with, my name is Stanley Fierstein, and I've lived in the city of Harrison practically all my life. Ten days ago I passed my eighty-seventh birthday, and for a man my age, I feel pretty good. I attribute this to the fact that I am quite active here in the Franklin Nursing Home, and I like to keep busy. And in that way I maintain the vitality, the strength, the vigor, everything that a human being needs to keep himself going day after day.

I was born in the city of Riga, the capital of Latvia. Now, Latvia was always an independent state. It's over toward the Black Sea. My parents . . . had, including myself, three children, and I was the baby. When they decided to come to the good old USA—and landed in Ellis Island in New York—I was 3 months old. So I can't tell you anything about Riga or Latvia or anything about Europe because I wasn't old enough to remember, and of course I often bragged when I grew older that when I came over on the ship, I didn't get seasick! And I make a joke out of it.

We moved to Harrison and I lived in Harrison for about fifty years. We lived in the north end of the city. . . . During my first semester of high school, my father became ill and passed away at a very young age of 40. I was a little over 14 years of age. Originally when we came here, we were very poor, and I had to go to work. My mother raised, all told, six children, three boys and three girls.

And I worked in a department store doing office work because I felt that I was more inclined toward mental work than I was toward physical work. I felt that I never would be a carpenter or a plumber or an electrician or anything that took strength or physical work. But

[25]

with my mind, I felt that I could always add well, and I loved mathematics. Before I knew it, the war came on, on April 6 in 1917, when the United States declared war. In September, I couldn't wait any longer, and I enlisted in the United States Navy.

I was assigned to the USS P—. That was a mine sweeper, and every day we used to go out sweeping the mines across the Atlantic and pick up what mines had been laid by the enemies and what dummy mines we could pick up that were laid by the United States Navy for practice purposes so we would know how to handle these things if any should come up from the water. I served on two different mine sweepers, and I served on a light ship. And I served on a submarine. And after the Armistice was signed I became an instructor with eighty-six or eighty-seven pupils.

After I was discharged, . . . I went back to my old job again, but this time not as an office clerk but as a salesman in a department store selling carpets. And to this day I hold the record as a salesman for earning more money in that store than anybody else since the store has been in existence. And I was complimented not only by the board of directors and the officers of the store, but the owner himself called me into his office and congratulated me for earning this particular amount of money. And in those days it was a lot of money, because, you know, when you earned $25.00 a week in those days that was a lot of money. But they raised me to $30.00 a week. The congratulations that I received was for earning $254 a week for four solid weeks for the amount of business that I brought in to that store.

In the meantime I met my sweetheart and we kept company for a couple of years, and she urged me to leave the store and go into business for myself. I knew a lot of people; I wasn't a backward citizen of any kind. I was always in the forefront, I always could meet any kind of a challenge, and speak on any subject because I was a great reader. On any subject, it made no difference, whether it was about the war, if it was national or international, state or local politics, anything, I was always interested in reading the events of the world. I married my sweetheart two years after I came home from the service. It was a wonderful marriage. I lost her after forty-two years of happiness, of love! [sobs] We never had one argument. We loved each other as if we were just beginning to court each other. The children she bore and which I fathered, they were so good. My wife gave them such a wonderful bringing up that I will use a Jewish phrase: I kvelled for my children because they were good, kind, considerate, they loved their parents and they obeyed. My word was law and their mother's word was law, and to this very day, after my wife passed away, my children still love me, respect me, and do everything I ask of them, just so that I am happy.

In Riga, my father had a big farm of his own, and he toiled every day on the soil, and he liked it very much, and so on. My mother had a brother here who was very well-to-do. When we came over, he put my father to work for him. My father worked for his brother-in-law, so to speak, till such time that he decided to go into business for himself. It was metals and rags. Junk business and all that sort of thing. And one time when things got slow, and he closed his business, he worked for another company. He got taken sick from working there—from all the rust that got down in his lungs—and he had to quit there, and he finally went back into his original business—metals and iron and scrap and all. Only my father was a small potato compared to my uncle, who used to buy and bale and ship carloads all over the country, my uncle did. He was a fine fellow. When we came over, we had nothing, and he provided us with a way of life until we got on our feet. He was very very good to us.

We very seldom talked about the past. At that time there were pogroms going on over there, and it was something we didn't care to talk about. It brought up memories that hurt us more inside than what good it would do to talk about it. None of us ever spoke about it.

I can go on and on and tell you more of various events of my life. But I don't know how much more I can talk about it because it seems that I'm bragging more than anything else—and that I don't want to do—and I don't want you to misconstrue me in telling you these things—that I'm bragging or telling you what a big shot I am, or this or that. It's nothing of the kind. My whole life has always been to help the next fellow—no matter how tough things may go for you, there's always someone that's worse off than you are.

[27]

[2]

Background and Context

The numbers and proportions of elderly people in the United States and other Western countries have been increasing rapidly. Whereas in 1870 the population of the United States included only 2 percent who were 65 years of age or older, the proportion had increased to over 11 percent by 1981 (Aronson and Shield 1982). Of the twenty million Americans over 65 in 1970, 35 percent were between the ages of 65 and 69, 27 percent between 70 and 74 years old, and 38 percent over the age of 75 (Vladeck 1980). Estimates of future proportions of the elderly in the United States population range from 15 percent in the next few decades (Leaf 1973) to 25 percent by the year 2020 (Butler 1975). And given the large gains made in public health and advances in science, life expectancy has increased from 49 years in 1900–1902 to 71.9 years in 1974 (Siegel 1978). Furthermore, the oldest segment of the United States population (the frail elderly) has increased the greatest amount (Rosenwaike and Dolinsky 1987).

These percentages are in sharp contrast to those of non-Western nations. Dependency ratios, which compare the population below age 15 plus those above age 65 with the population between ages 15 and 64, illustrate some of the difference between countries. In Asia, there are approximately 90–100 individuals in the productive years for every one individual living beyond age 80; in Africa, the ratio is 75:1; and in the United States and Western Europe, the ratio is only 30:1 (Aronson and Shield 1982). As good nutrition, better disease prevention, and advances in medical research have created an extended life expectancy, there are more frail elderly (over the age of 75) who live with multiple physical ailments so that "the elderly are not only the most frequently ill, but also the most seriously ill" (Leaf 1982:366).

The Nursing Home Population

Of the twenty-three million people in the United States over the age of 65, between three and four million need help from family, friends, or social agencies (Ball 1977). Most nursing-home residents have no relatives. At any given time 95 percent of the nation's elderly live in the community and 5 percent are in institutions (Kayser-Jones 1981). Many nursing-home residents are discharged back to the community and therefore do not die in the nursing home. Indeed, Liu and Manton (1983) conducted a prospective study of nursing home admissions which showed that a high percentage of residents had short stays, most being discharged within one year. Their data is based on recent Department of Health, Education, and Welfare statistics (National Center for Health Statistics 1979). Liu and Manton also found that "nursing homes are not simply terminal care facilities for long- or short-term patients. What is perhaps most notable is the strong inverse relationship between the LOS [length of stay] and the likelihood of dying in the facility. Clearly a type of inertia is operating such that, once a patient has resided in the nursing home for more than a year, he is likely to remain there until his death" (1984:72). According to Vladeck (1980), the average length of stay is 2.6 years: "More than a quarter stay more than three years, and another third stay one to three years. In the oxymoronic language favored by health administrators, 30 percent of all nursing-home discharges are due to death; most of the others are sent either to general hospitals (often to prevent the embarrassment of having the resident die in the nursing home itself) or to other nursing homes (generally for financial reasons). Some small proportion of nursing-home patients receive rehabilitative services of adequate intensity to permit their returning home; another small, but uncounted, proportion simply cannot stand the nursing home and leave. Most remain until or through the acute episode that eventually kills them" (1980:16–17). Eighty-four percent of nursing-home residents are 75 years of age or older. The typical nursing-home resident is female, 80 years old, white, and widowed. Whereas 59 percent of the general population over 65 is female, in nursing homes over 72

[29]

percent of the residents are female. The number of people in nursing homes has tripled in the last two decades, and most of this increase can be attributed to the fact that the population over age 75 has nearly doubled since 1960 (Vladeck 1980).

In analyzing admissions and lengths of stay, researchers cite difficulties in projecting accurate utilization patterns. For example, Faulwell and Pomerantz (1981) have shown that older physicians institutionalize their patients less readily than younger physicians do. Additionally, when there are more cultural factors in common between the physician and the patient, the likelihood of a recommendation to institutionalize is reduced. Wingard, Jones, and Kaplan (1987) have noted that researchers compare different factors and utilize varying definitions in their analyses. A few useful generalizations can be made, however. (1) Whereas 4–5 percent of the population 65 and older live in long-term care facilities, approximately 20 percent of the population over 65 die in nursing homes. This figure is due in part to the fact that many people are transferred to nursing homes just prior to death. (2) The risk of institutionalization increases with age. (3) Women have a higher risk of institutionalization than men largely because they live longer. (4) The availability of care givers (usually a wife) delays or avoids institutionalization. (5) A person's functional status, that is, the ability to perform activities of daily living (ADL), is a more reliable predictor than the kinds of illnesses or disabilities that an individual may have.

A History of Nursing Homes

Beginning in the seventeenth century in England, hospitals excluded obstetrical, indigent, and insane patients, as well as lepers and children (Freymann 1974). Primarily shelters, their medical function was incidental at the start, and patients usually had to pay a burial deposit before being admitted. American hospitals were modeled on these English institutions, which restricted their purview to a narrow segment of the population that had certain acute and episodic diseases. The early Christian belief that linked the poor and the sick with a nearness to God gave way to a Puritan belief that equated disease and poverty with a deserved moral state.

The aged and indigent were housed outside hospitals, and work was incorporated into their regime. These poorhouses proliferated. Updike's (1958) novel *The Poorhouse Fair* describes both the antagonism between the inmates and the prefect who manages the poorhouse and the isolation of the poorhouse from the rest of the community. The townspeople see the poorhouse population only at the time of the fair. Then the inmates are on display, as it were, selling crafts for revenue, in a circuslike spectacle. Cut off from the community, the poorhouse seems timeless: "They [the townspeople] felt the poorhouse would always be there, exempt from time. That some residents died, and others came, did not occur to them; a few believed that the name of the prefect was still Mendelssohn. In a sense the poorhouse would indeed outlast their homes. The old continue to be old-fashioned, though their youths were modern. We grow backward, aging into our father's opinions and even into those of our grandfathers" (1958:112).

Poorhouses were common until the 1930s. Social Security legislation of the 1930s stipulated that only those patients receiving temporary care in hospitals were eligible for state support. Therefore inmates of public institutions remained excluded, and noninstitutional care was rewarded. As Thomas (1969) has described, proprietary (for profit) nursing homes were begun because of federal legislation in 1935 that reimbursed care given outside institutions, preferably in the home (outdoor relief). This policy was in contrast to the previous philosophy that the poor and indigent could receive care only in almshouses and only as charity. Private homes and boarding houses were accepted as nonpublic institutions following the Social Security act of 1935 and could be reimbursed by the government. The result has been that whereas the number of public nursing-home beds has barely increased since 1935, by 1963, 86 percent of nursing-home beds were proprietary (Freymann 1974:32).

Funding

The inception of third-party payments was based on two principles that underlay hospital functioning. Hospitals charged by the day, and doctors were paid for each service performed (Freymann 1974). With the economic hardship caused by the Depression of the 1930s, few patients could pay, and hospitals were threatened by bankruptcy. The start of Blue Shield in 1939 rescued hospitals by reimbursing doctors for the work they performed within hospitals. The principles underly-

[31]

ing funding mechanisms in operation today are fundamentally the same.

The Social Security Act of 1935 provided a federal program offering to states matching grants-in-aid called Old Age Assistance (OAA). This program was considered to be temporary; it was assumed that Social Security would eventually obviate the necessity for OAA. Because of the bad reputation of almshouses, this legislation also ensured that public funds not be used for public institutions. Cash relief, left to the discretion of the recipients, was considered preferable. Most of the institutionalized aged still needed indoor relief, however, and this need spurred the growth of private nursing homes.

Following the growth of hospitals permitted by the 1946 Hill-Burton Act, nursing homes benefited from subsidies given to those homes that operated in conjunction with hospitals.

Social Security legislation was amended in 1965 to include Medicare and Medicaid (Title XVIII and Title XIX). Medicare was to pay for hospital services for those over age 65 needing up to one hundred days of recuperative care following an acute hospitalization of at least three days. Medicaid extended medical coverage to all, regardless of age, who were medically indigent. It was to be administered by the states for skilled nursing care.[1]

By 1969, nursing homes receiving federal reimbursement were required to have at least one full-time registered nurse. In 1970, Medicaid standards for nursing homes were relaxed because most homes in the United States could not meet the requirements that had been set for skilled nursing facilities. To bring all nursing homes up to standard was expensive. The Miller Amendment of 1970 created the system of Intermediate Care Facilities, whose residents did not need skilled nursing care. Lower staffing standards were considered appropriate for these facilities.[2]

Public outrage over several tragic nursing-home incidents in the early 1970s provoked the Nixon administration to implement standards enforcement. Since 1974, reimbursement for skilled nursing and intermediate care facilities has come under Medicaid and reimbursement for skilled nursing care under Medicare. The highest reimbursement by Medicare and Medicaid is for skilled care. Nursing homes are licensed according to whether they provide skilled nursing care, intermediate care, or some combination of both.[3] To qualify for funding, licensed facilities must follow state and federal regulations that mandate physician services, nursing services, medical records, rehabilitative services, dietetic services, and quality assurance. The regulations stipulate the number of staff required and their educational standards.

In recent years the implementation of diagnostic-related groups (DGRs) has had a significant impact on nursing homes. Hospitals are reimbursed according to particular formulas that key to specific diseases. Each disease is worth a certain number of days and a certain amount of reimbursement. One important effect of this policy has been to discharge elderly patients from hospitals earlier than before. As a result, they leave the hospital sicker than they used to and enter the nursing home in worse condition.

The Jews of Harrison

The first Jews who came to Harrison between 1840 and 1880 were primarily peddlers from Germany. By 1900, there were approximately sixteen hundred Jewish names in the Harrison city directory, about 1 percent of the city's population.[4] From 1880 until World War I, there was a rapid growth in the Jewish population. Most of the new Jewish immigrants came from Eastern Europe and were less prosperous than their German predecessors. The majority were young men escaping military service or the horrors of the Russian raids on Jews, the pogroms. During this period self-help organizations in Harrison settled and aided the poorer immigrants. Temples sprang up in the various neighborhoods and reflected the local languages and customs of the native communities.

Near the turn of the century, a Jewish women's group in Harrison was formed to help settle immigrants. When it was discovered that a Jewish man had died in the state almshouse and had been improperly buried, the women determined to provide a place to care for the needy Jewish elderly and to ensure that they were buried according to prescribed Jewish ritual and law. The women rented a house, and incorporated the Franklin Nursing Home shortly thereafter. A husband and wife served as caretakers for the home; they made the meals and saw to the needs of the residents.

The Franklin Nursing Home purchased land in the 1930s, and a new building was constructed for the two dozen residents. The explicit philosophy of the Franklin Nursing Home had changed by this time: the Jewish elderly were now thought to need not only shelter

[33]

and kosher food, but activities, medical care, and religious ceremonies. Sicker residents were admitted, and the nursing home's census gradually increased. Over the years new construction enabled
more people to be admitted, including wealthy people who needed
the services of the nursing home. By the early 1980s the Jewish population of the Harrison area was estimated at eighteen thousand. Over
two hundred residents now live in the Franklin Nursing Home, and a
daycare center on the premises provides supportive services to elderly
in the community.

The Franklin Nursing Home

The Franklin Nursing Home facility comprises a new main building
and the older, smaller wing. One enters the new building today
through automatic doors opening on a lounge and a reception desk.
On the first floor are administrative, social-worker, and nursing of-
fices, a large meeting room for parties and meetings, a chapel, a hair
salon, an occupational therapy room, a physical therapy room, and
dental, podiatric, and opthalmic clinics. Above the first floor are four
resident floors, with predominantly double rooms. Three of these
floors connect to the three floors of the smaller wing, each of which
houses residents who are considered to be "self-care," that is, requiring less care than those in the new building. Almost all of the rooms in
the wing are single rooms. On each floor of the new building and the
wing there is a nurses' station and a resident dining room with a
refrigerator and a sink.

In the new building, four corridors fan out from the centrally located nurses' station. Near the nurses' station are the main elevators,
which are in use all day transporting residents to activities and
therapies on the first floor and back again. Two small lounge rooms are
located at either end of each floor of the new building. These are used
for staff members on breaks and for private family visits. On each
corridor is the bathing room and a closet for linens. Directly behind
the nurses' station is the locked medicine closet, a bathroom for staff,
and a small room in which staff members smoke and gossip during
breaks.

Because well more than half of the beds are licensed as skilled-
nursing-care beds, I call the Franklin Nursing Home a nursing home
rather than a home for the aged, which implies a higher level of

functioning of its residents. Eighty percent of the residents at Franklin receive Medicaid reimbursement. Medicaid reimbursement varies from facility to facility and depends on many factors. Franklin loses approximately twenty dollars per day for each Medicaid patient. This gap has remained more or less constant for the last decade or so. If a resident is hospitalized for three or more days and requires skilled nursing care (SN) following the hospitalization (for example, sterile dressings, registered nurse procedures, intravenous feedings), he or she becomes eligible for Medicare for the next one hundred days in the nursing home as a skilled care patient. If skilled care is required for more than one hundred days, then the patient is covered by Medicaid. Medicaid pays for those intermediate care residents (ICF I and ICF II) who are deemed financially needy. Care status also determines the physical placement of the resident within the home. In general, the 14 percent of residents who are able to care for themselves with minimal supervision (ICF II) are placed in the self-care unit of the wing. They are expected to be ambulatory and in little need of nurses. They lead fairly independent lives within the constraints of the nursing home. In the new building the sickest residents requiring twenty-four-hour skilled nursing care (SN) are on the second and third floors. The 25 percent of healthier residents requiring less nursing care (ICF I) are usually placed on the remaining three floors. They need twenty-four-hour supervision by nursing personnel and nursing assistants and orderlies, though they do not require skilled nursing care. Exceptions to this pattern of resident placement are made in order to lighten the work load on certain floors: residents who need less care are sometimes placed on the second and third floors so that the nursing work required is not as extensive as it otherwise might be.

Staff

There were over 250 staff members at Franklin at the time of my fieldwork. The predominantly white and female staff consists of administrators, registered nurses (RNs), nursing assistants, orderlies, maintenance staff, dietary staff, housekeepers, social workers, and occupational and recreational therapists. Union workers are licensed practical nurses (LPNs), nursing assistants, orderlies, maintenance staff, dietary staff, and housekeepers, or approximately 75 percent of Franklin employees.

The nursing staff includes the director of nurses, the nursing supervisors, and the director of in-training. There were 22 RNs, 28 LPNs, and 110 nursing assistants and orderlies at the time of my fieldwork. On each floor of the new building there is at least one RN, one LPN, and several nursing assistants and orderlies for the day shift (7:00 A.M. to 3:00 P.M.). For the evening and night shifts (from 3:00 P.M. to 11:00 P.M. and from 11:00 P.M. to 7:00 A.M.) there are usually no RNs on duty, and the staffing requirements in general are less stringent. On each floor in the wing there is usually one RN and one LPN on duty during the day and one LPN on duty during the evening and night shifts. Staffing ratios on each shift are higher than what is required by state regulations. No training was required of nursing assistants and orderlies; however, just recently, a nursing-assistant training program on the premises of Franklin was begun.

Until the late 1970s, the Social Service Department consisted of one part-time social worker. Since then, the Social Service Department has had at least one full-time social worker and several part-time social work students or social worker assistants. The Franklin staff includes a part-time medical director and a consulting psychiatrist. Medical students rotate through the facility for gerontology and community health electives. The physical therapist and occupational therapist each has at least one assistant.

Though pay scales at Franklin are higher than at other nursing homes in the area, there is continual and increasing difficulty recruiting and holding staff members, which reflects the shortage of nursing-home employees throughout the country. Though a core of staff members stay at Franklin for some length of time, there is increasing dependence upon nursing pools. Perhaps one-quarter to one-third of the staff is made up from pools, depending on the particular shift. In addition, within the last decade there have been several threatened strikes, including one near miss during my fieldwork. A month-long strike occurred in the mid-1980s.

Ethnic diversity marks Harrison, and this diversity is somewhat reflected in the staff makeup. Though the staff is mostly white, there are a large number of blacks (African and American) and some Indochinese, many Portuguese, and some Caribbean staff members. The administrators, the social workers, and the medical staff are distinguished socioeconomically from the lower-paid and lower-status housekeepers, nurses, nursing assistants, and orderlies. Religious distinctions among staff are important too, especially considering the fact that the clientele is almost exclusively Jewish. Of all the staff members employed at Franklin while I was conducting fieldwork, no more than a dozen were Jewish, and they occupied administrative and social-work positions.

Voice: Max Sager

My father met my mother for the first time on the day they were married. They were both from Russia.

I don't know the names of the villages they came from, but when they heard one day that the Cossacks were on a drunken rampage, they knew it was time for them to leave because they would be killed. So they sold the pittance that they had, and they used their few bucks to get to a place from which they sailed to America.

I seldom saw my parents. My father would open the store at two in the morning. He'd go down to the cellar and make some sort of drink that you would sell with soda water in it. It was expensive. It was three cents. But if you only had a penny or two cents—you've heard the expression "two cents plain"? That's what it means. Two cents plain.

After my parents died I didn't have a nickle. The only thing my father was interested in were the Jewish holidays. He'd close the goddamn' candy store and go to shul. You know what a shul is? And spend all day, every minute. Of course, my mother couldn't do that because at an orthodox shul the women didn't amount to a row of beans. They had to climb a flight of rusty stairs and get some sort of seat. Sometimes they could hear; most times they couldn't. The men were the bosses. I went with my father. After we got to the shul, after five minutes, I did what all the other kids do. There was a big playground. We went out and we played. All the kids played. [Later, with the couple who cared for me], *I went to a thing called Ethical Culture Society. Have you ever heard of it? I was one of them, one of those.*

[The couple, Jennie and Samuel F., was very rich and knew every-

[38]

one in the art world.] *On Saturday afternoons when someone famous would come, Jennie wanted to know in advance what I would like* [to eat]. *And that's what we'd have. Occasionally, the butler would pull me aside and say, "For gosh sakes, don't you ever eat?" "Of course, I want borscht and I want lox, all the Jewish dishes," and they were not mean about it at all, but they were really surprised that I would never ask about an ingredient or a meal that they knew about. With five butlers Jennie and Samuel didn't find it difficult to get things. They'd pick up one of the phones and say, "This is Samuel F. calling and I want this," and in five minutes you'd get it. Unless it was something that came right from Europe. I was never adopted by this family but I lived with them. Jennie always said, "Come, come, and change your name. You're my son." I said, "Look, I appreciate everything. I think you're a wonderful person, but please. My mother was my mother. I hardly knew her, but I will not do anything to disrespect her. I could not do this. I will always be what I am, and if my name is changed, okay, for the public or your friends, it's changed, but I'm always Max, and my name is Sager." And they did respect it. Although sometimes we'd sit upstairs in the library—the library was almost as big as the one in New York!—and we'd sit there and she'd come in every five minutes: "Would you like some tea? Strawberries? Would you like—" you know. Real motherly. Because . . . to them . . . they were my parents, and to them, I was their child. Actually, I never felt that way.*

When I went to the private school, I was right in the heart of the Italian district, and around me were people who either had been to reform school or jail or who were going to get there very shortly. One boy was a violinist—he used to practice at the school. He came and he practiced. He came back an hour later, after he had drunk his wine. This particular day, he didn't come back! When it was two hours, we were a little concerned, so we called him. He had dropped dead. We don't know why. We went to [this boy's] *church, and I took it for granted that I was going to go, and so did everybody, all my friends. But the nuns would not allow it. They didn't want me to come because I was Jewish. His sister took the nuns aside, but, well, I could tell from the expression on their faces what they were saying. They said, "No, we're sorry, we can't do it, because if we do we'll be thrown out of where we're staying as nuns." How do you like that? But for three days there was eating and drinking and flowers! They came in all sizes. It was macabre. One set of flowers was a violin, only it was as large as a cello, all made out of flowers. And everyone was drinking. Drinking, drinking, drinking. That was their way of showing respect and love.*

I felt more at home in the F. family because Jennie was Jewish even though they didn't practice anymore. But I didn't really feel at home. For instance, they wanted to give me a birthday party. Who shall I invite? What shall we do? What sort of a party shall it be? What shall we drink? What shall we eat? Well, I told them all the things I thought my friends would like. It was the most boring thing in the world because first of all, when my friends got to the place and they saw what it looked like, and here was this stuffed shirt opening the door for them, they didn't feel at home! I said, "Come on. Come on—this is a party." But it wasn't. I couldn't do anything about it. [Jennie and Mr. F.] were heartbroken—Jennie, my so-called mother. Mr. F. was a little more realistic. He expected that. That's what happened. The kids sat there as though they were at reform school, and when it came time to eat something, they looked from one to another—What do ya eat with a knife or a fork? When do you use the napkins? That sort of thing. It made me uncomfortable. And then Jennie came up with a brilliant idea which was the stupidest of all: "Recite a poem for them." How was I going to make them feel at home? So I told some sort of corny joke and got out of that. Okay.

[The F. family] went to Maine for the summers, but I didn't go. Two of the servants stayed with me, and the other three took care of them. Of course I needed servants. What would I have done without them? What the hell. I couldn't go to the bathroom without them. And it's surprising how often [Jennie and Samuel would] come home. They found excuses; they wanted to be with me all the time. And I felt hemmed in. How about your suit? Look, you haven't bought a suit! Go down—where shall we go? I said, "Let me alone, will you?" I could be nasty as hell. They let me alone. It got to the point, they were afraid I'd just get up and they'd never see me again.

It's just like the play Annie. I haven't seen it, but the story is something like the female version of my life. Here's the kid. And this multimillionaire who suddenly gets it in his mind he's going to adopt somebody. That was I. To me they seemed about 110, but they were probably about 50. My parents were young when they died. My mother must have been in her early thirties and my father was about the same age. Oh yes. I had an uncle and an aunt. They were truly my uncle and my aunt. They wouldn't have come to see me because well, they wouldn't. Even I would have been ashamed—their language was atrocious, they didn't even speak English. But occasionally I'd go there. They'd invite me to come and stay over. And the next morning, my aunt would say to me, "I have a present for you." And do you know what she gave me? Three pennies. Three pennies. I thought it was the greatest gift I'd ever gotten in my life. And every Friday they would come to our home when my mother was alive and my father. They'd play poker. And I loved those Fridays for another reason. It was the night when we used to have the delicatessen. And there was a German bakery nearby. German cakes. And we'd have Jewish delicatessen. And boy, they'd play for heavy stakes. Two cents. I'll raise you a cent! He'd be there for an hour, studying his cards. Ah, I raise you two cents more. So that's it. I got to stay up and eat all of the delicatessen. I loved that stuff. I still do.

[3]

Residents

Franklin residents come from different countries, have worked in a variety of occupations, practice Judaism in individual fashion, have undergone and withstood specific circumstances in individual ways, and have been admitted to the nursing home for different reasons. No resident knows all other residents, and most knew only a few before admission. A number of the residents are related to each other. In addition to several husband-wife pairs, there are also siblings, cousins, and even a few parent-child combinations. The heterogeneity of this group is maintained within the walls of the nursing home at the same time that a leveling of status occurs because of the necessity for admission.

Resident Profile

Admission to Franklin used to require that the applicant be physically able to walk over the threshold. Now the residents are older and more frail, reflecting a general aging Jewish population nationally (Rosenwaike 1986). The average age on entry to Franklin has risen for both males and females. In 1970, the average age of males was 80.0 and of females, 78.2. By 1982, the ages had risen to 85.3 and 83.2 (Clinton, Shield, and Aronson 1983).

Females have always outnumbered males in the nursing home, as in most nursing homes, and the proportion of females rose from 62.4 percent at the beginning of the 1970s to 69.1 percent in 1982. Because females live in the home an average of 2.1 years longer than males do, the actual ratio of females to males as reflected in annual census records of the home is greater than the admission proportion indicates. In 1970–73, the July 1 census averaged 71.2 percent females, and by 1978–82, the proportion of females had risen to 73.5 percent. While the average duration of stay for males seems to be decreasing somewhat, the average length of stay for females is increasing slightly. At present the average duration of stay per female is 4.6 years in contrast to 3.7 years for males, even though a sizable number of residents die soon after admission (as in many nursing homes). Overall, these figures represent longer lengths of stay than those in other nursing homes.

The fact of a steadily increasing age upon admission for both males and females may be due to the daycare center located at Franklin, which delays admission to the nursing home for some. Increased frailty of new admissions seems to be due not only to greater age but to the effect of diagnostic-related groups in hospitals, which often results in patients' leaving hospitals prematurely and entering nursing homes rather than returning to the community.

Another change is the percentage of residents with Alzheimer's disease (SDAT, or senile dementia of the Alzheimer's type), the most predominant form of dementing illness in the aged. Determining numbers of cases is difficult because of problems in differential diagnoses (Shore 1983).[1] According to the director of social services, at least half of the Franklin residents during my fieldwork exhibited some kind of enduring and progressive dementia or confusion (see Table 1).

The incidence of dementia rises steeply with age and shows a higher ratio of severely afflicted men to women than expected.

Table 1. Residents with dementia

Under age 80	Males	Females
No sign of dementia	4	12
Mild dementia	2	9
Moderate dementia	5	4
Severe dementia	3	7
Over age 80		
No sign of dementia	16	48
Mild dementia	9	27
Moderate dementia	6	36
Severe dementia	21	43

[43]

Table 2. Goldfarb mental status test

1. Where are we now?
2. Where is this place located?
3. What is today's date? What is the day of the month?
4. What month is it?
5. What year is it?
6. How old are you?
7. What is your birth date?
8. What year were you born?
9. Who is the president of the United States?
10. Who was the president before him?

Testing for dementia is problematic. The most accurate tests take time to administer, but few residents are able to tolerate lengthy tests. Definitive diagnosis of SDAT can be made only on autopsy. The Goldfarb scale, regularly used at the nursing home, consists of ten basic questions (see Table 2).

The accuracy of the test in determining and differentiating dementia is probably minimal. The Goldfarb is usually administered at the time of admission or in the first week of residence, a time often marked by confusion, disorientation, and unhappiness at having been admitted. There is no provision for readministering it three months after admission when considerable adjustment to the nursing home may reasonably be expected to have taken place. Subjective interpretations of answers constitute another problem. For example, in response to the question about the last president, one resident could not recall the name exactly, but said he was "Jimmy, the peanut man." The social worker did not know whether to consider her response correct or not. Another person, when asked today's date, got up and went over to his calendar to look, refusing to agree to the rule that he know the date without looking. The social worker decided that he "got an A for effort" and considered him intact. Valid test results are also impeded when the person has mood disorders or sensory deficits (such as being unable to hear the questions).

Backgrounds

The majority of the residents immigrated to this country from Eastern Europe or Russia at the beginning of the twentieth century. Many joined relatives who were already established in Harrison. Some came with siblings and parents; others came by themselves, or with one sibling, or with one parent. A significant minority came to Harrison following World War II, and they form a separate group within the home. More recent Russian immigrants have been admitted to Franklin in the last decades. Another segment was born in this country.

A large number of the nursing-home population came to the United States with little or no money and established small businesses; others worked in textile and jewelry factories, peddled junk, automotive parts, fruits and vegetables, were liquor salesmen, shoe salesmen, furniture dealers, or haberdashers. The women took various jobs usually until they married. A few of the women were fashion models; others were saleswomen and factory workers, and many were partners with their husbands in small businesses. Some residents are well educated and were in teaching and other white-collar and professional occupations before retirement. The socioeconomic status of the residents varies considerably as a result. Many were considered successful and lived affluently in the years before admission, and others occupied much more modest positions in the community.

Although the literature on aging indicates that most people who enter nursing homes do not have children or other family members, most Franklin residents were married and are currently widowed, have siblings, and many have children. A large number have siblings, spouses, or children who live nearby. As Goldstein and Goldscheider (1968) and Goldstein (1981) have stressed, Jewish fertility rates have traditionally been low. Rates were especially low during the Depression when couples limited family size because of meager financial resources. This is probably one of the reasons that a significant number (though not the majority) of residents at Franklin have one child or no children. Having few or no children raises one's chances of entering a nursing home, for one of the major options of support is removed.

Many residents' children live locally. Like other old people in the United States, the residents prefer living with a spouse, or alone, rather than with adult children. Most often, the entering resident was married and had lived with his or her spouse until the spouse's death. Deteriorating health, loneliness, fear of neighborhood crime, and similar considerations often lead the elderly person to live with one of the adult children, usually a daughter.

[45]

Reasons for Admission

Admission to the nursing home can result from any of a variety of factors. Because increasing numbers of women now work, the aged parent in the adult child's home is often alone and lonely. With the greater age of the entire population, care-giving children are frequently in their sixties or older. This "generation in the middle" (Neugarten 1968, 1979) is encountering medical problems and may still be financially helping their own offspring. The aged parent, often frail and beset with multiple chronic ailments, requires increasing care. A family may initiate application to the nursing home when one or more of these factors are present. Actual admission may occur a few years later, after a precipitating incident such as a hospitalization.[2]

Many residents are admitted after the spouse has died. Inadequacy of community resources, such as sheltered housing and convenient, inexpensive transportation, propel an elderly person into the nursing home where aids for daily living are provided. Though Americans are loathe to institutionalize their aged family members, as gerontologists (especially Brody 1985) have repeatedly shown, many elderly cannot be managed at home, Alzheimer's disease being a prime reason. Furthermore, many nursing-home residents with family have alienated them (Retsinas 1986). Their relationships have always been strained, and they remain problematic within the nursing home as well. The following brief portraits are of some of the varied residents who served as subjects and informants.

Some of the Residents

Bessie Curtin. Bessie Curtin, 81, was born in a neighboring city and lived there until she married. Her husband died years ago. Her oldest daughter lives locally and was the one who pushed for her admission to Franklin. Mrs. Curtin had been calling her as often as thirty times a day. Mrs. Curtin has had several psychiatric hospitalizations in the past, and the daughter felt her mother was out of control. Now that she is in the nursing home, Mrs. Curtin complains about how much it costs, and she says she will move to Florida. A number of residents have complained about her in the few weeks since she has been in the nursing home. She has no serious medical problems, but the daughter could not handle her and felt that she could not live on her own.

[46]

Leo Feldman. He was born in Russia in 1899. At 12, he was a boxmaker and came to the United States during the Russian Revolution to avoid conscription. He has several medical problems, including arteriosclerotic heart disease, deafness, and difficulties resulting from a colostomy performed because of colon cancer. He is forgetful, and the social worker thinks that if his wife were somewhat stronger he might be manageable at home. The recent death of their daughter was a tremendous blow to them both. His wife is on the waiting list for Franklin and is having difficulty visiting her husband because of the ten-dollar round-trip cab fare.

Fannie Luden. She had been in the daycare program, but became increasingly anxious and suffered various anxiety attacks. She is a diabetic who does not follow her diet. Her other medical problems are arteriosclerotic heart disease, senile dementia (based on the Goldfarb test), and a history of fainting spells. She had lived in housing for the elderly, but she was having accidents that resulted in weekly trips to the emergency room. Since she entered Franklin, she has seemed much less anxious; she sleeps through the night and expresses satisfaction with her life.

Sarah Tessler. A "young-looking 90," she was born in Latvia and emigrated to the United States when she was a little girl. She was a salesperson and was married and divorced quite early. One of her sisters lives in Franklin. She seems to be quite demented. She was admitted five years ago after repeatedly leaving pots on the hot stove and showing other signs of confusion. Quiet, she loses her train of thought midsentence, participates in some of the activities, and generally gets along with her roommate, who is also confused. Staff members say that she whines when she cannot find her room.

Norman Klein. He is 89 years old and was admitted 10 years ago "so that I can be among Jews." He was born in Kiev; both parents died before he was 5; he was raised by his sister. He emigrated to the United States as a teenager, became a tailor, married, had three children, and led a comfortable life. His wife died a year before he was admitted. Two of his children live nearby. Though he is somewhat alert, he scored three correct out of ten on the Goldfarb. Most important, he is blind and very anxious. He stays in his room by himself most of the time. Though he goes to physical therapy, his arms are severely contracted and he can walk only a short distance. He has a mild case of diabetes.

Sam Krakow. Sam Krakow, 85 years old, had been successful in business and was admitted to Franklin ten years ago after his wife died and he had numerous blackouts and could not be left alone. His medical problems include dementia, cataracts, arteriosclerotic heart disease, peptic ulcer disease, chronic obstructive pulmonary disease, and some deafness. Though his sister lives nearby, she apparently does not visit. His brother lives locally but also does not visit. Staff members say he is severely demented and is constantly making sexual remarks and trying to grab them. From his case history it is unclear how many of his problems were present at the time of admission and how many developed afterward. He can perform almost no activities of daily living.

Max Sager. One of the nursing home's younger residents, he is only 78 years of age. He is a fastidious and handsome man who seemed to age visibly over the course of fieldwork. He was once a sculptor and studied in Berlin in the mid-1930s, innocently undisturbed by the rise of Hitler. He grew up in a nearby city and, except for his stay in Berlin, has always lived in the United States. His personal story, including orphanhood at an early age, is painful for him to relate. A wealthy philanthropic couple who was unable to have children wanted to adopt him, and subsidized his education. Feeling lonely and deprived amidst wealth and the obvious love of his would-be adoptive parents, he wished he could have been just like other children. His only child, a son, married a non-Jew and died recently.

He has had several medical and psychiatric hospitalizations in recent years, and as a result his room in the nursing home has been changed several times. Residents refer to him as aloof, acting better than them, and crazy. He reads and is interested in political events and art. At times he feels he is in danger in the nursing home and that he has enemies. Recently he has become quite weak, depressed, withdrawn, and frightened.

Helena Grosz. When she was 86 years old, she was admitted to the nursing home without knowing that her stay was to be permanent. She had been living in an apartment near her son's family, but the family felt she could not live on her own any longer. It is unclear whether Mrs. Grosz wanted to live with her son's family, but it was evident that they were unwilling to consider that alternative. Whereas she had been involved in outside activities earlier, she became withdrawn and sullen and refused to go out.

Mrs. Grosz emigrated from Czechoslavakia after World War II. Her husband and her older sons had died in the war. She remarried and came to the United States and was widowed again. During my fieldwork, when she was newly admitted, she was angry at the son near whom she had been living and was comparing him unfavorably with her son who lives in another state. Her "bad" son believed that she must be in a protected environment because she was found once on the floor, having fainted, and on numerous occasions she has burned herself with cigarettes.

Though Mrs. Grosz thinks she is to return home, her family does not know how to tell her that Franklin is now home. She refuses to decorate her room with belongings from her former apartment or take more clothes or make friends. She insists upon smoking wherever and whenever she pleases. Though cigarettes have been confiscated from her, she manages to secure them somehow, baffling the staff. She wants nothing to do with anyone in the nursing home and says she does not belong here. She seemed confused and disoriented when she was admitted, but she became oriented soon thereafter.

According to her son, she used to sing beautifully, but before admission refused to sing at all. The staff surmised that she was unwilling to sing because her standards were too high. A staff goal was that she be encouraged to sing once more.

Stanley Fierstein. He looks younger than his 87 years. He prides himself on his fancy clothing and his vitality. He says that he admitted himself to the nursing home after the lingering death of his wife following her stroke several years earlier because he did not want to burden his children, all of whom live within one hour away. He dislikes living in the nursing home; he feels that he has no privacy, the rules are too restrictive, the female residents are shrill and possessive, and some of the staff members are not to his liking.

Having been in this country since he was an infant, he prides himself on his American-ness and scorns those in the nursing home who act foreign. In the Navy he encountered much anti-Semitism. He takes pleasure in recounting his accomplishments and those of his children, grandchildren, and great-grandchildren. He considers a woman whom he had known in high school and had remet at Franklin to be his girlfriend.

Mr. Fierstein has a reputation for being active and argumentative. He believes that his daily walks and constant activity keep him youthful. He resents that he is not allowed to drive, and says that if he were allowed to be on the board of trustees he could change many things, starting with a kitchen that would provide greater variety.

Bernice Meyerhov. She and her brother Isaac Grigor occupy the same room in the part of the building that is for the sicker residents. Mrs. Meyerhov seems extremely fragile and frail. She has fine features and a tiny body. She has little appetite, does not like the food, tries to eat, and has been losing weight steadily. She is the healthier of the two. She is 93 and her brother is a few years younger and senile. Mrs. Meyerhov was born and grew up in Russia. When she was married and had two children, she managed to survive the pogroms in Russia while her husband and two brothers were killed. She and her children struggled in Europe during World War I.

As was common among the Jewish orthodox, she married her uncle at her mother's urging. After this husband's death, she and her children emigrated to Puerto Rico, where she became fluent in Spanish. Since Bernice and Isaac moved to the United States, Isaac, a shoe salesman, helped Bernice in many ways, but a head injury was the beginning of severe mental problems for him. He turned from a generous and gentle man into an unpredictably provocative and irascible man.

In the nursing home Mrs. Meyerhov provides much of the care for her brother, who is twice her size and frequently combative. She refuses to have a separate room, believing it is her turn to help him. He is incontinent, and she helps him out of bed, day and night, to take him to the bathroom. Though she has been urged not to do such physical caring for him, she says that when she tells the nurses to help her, they take too long to come, so she does the work herself. She shrugs her shoulders at the difficulties of living in the nursing home, understanding that situations can be much worse. She has a Spanish-speaking aide who treats her kindly because Mrs. Meyerhov knows her language. With staff urging, she occasionally goes to bingo games in the lounge downstairs.

Sarah Zeldin. She jokes that if she married an Aby Abramovitz she would get her meal tray first and would not ever have to eat cold dinners again. Alphabetical rules typify for her the daily, petty annoyances of the nursing home. Eighty-three years old, Mrs. Zeldin entered the nursing home with her husband three years ago, and he died six months later. Though she misses him very much, she considers her situation to be fairly good overall.

She is in the minority of residents who were born in the United

States. She and her husband had no children. She is grateful to anyone who visits her because, without children, she has no one who "must" visit. She is scornful of those residents who complain that their children and grandchildren do not visit them because she feels they do not recognize how lucky they are to have family. Mrs. Zeldin likes some of the activities that the nursing home provides, and she is in reasonably good health. She talks acerbically, however, about the time-killing nature of the activities and about the nettlesome aspects of living in a place where the staff assumes the residents do not know quite what they mean.

Charlie Kassin. A young-looking 81, he is active and energetic. He and another resident, Helen Safrin, have been linked romantically. Other residents consider them an unlikely pair and think he is not good enough for her. He says he would never marry again because his children would object that he was showing disloyalty to their mother.

He was born in Russia and emigrated with a brother when he was in his teens. He worked as a plumbing supply salesman, married, and had several children. He liked to make deals and is proud of the fact that no one could push him around or trick him. He says that he entered the nursing home so that his children would not fight about which one of them would take him in. Some residents do not like him, claiming that he is dishonest. He argues with various staff members frequently. Nonetheless, he enjoys the activities and has various routines such as walking through the nursing home every morning greeting people and checking on several people he knows. He has an engaging style, talks proudly about his life and family, and appears satisfied with the present.

Freida Kleinberg. Freida Kleinberg, 85, was born in Russia and emigrated to the United States when she was 6 years old. When her seventh child was about to be born, her husband died. She had to place three of her children in an orphanage because she could not take care of all of them. After visiting them every week for several years, she was finally able to take them out and support them.

She was admitted because of a number of health problems. She is very thin and tells the staff that what she would really like is some cherrystone clams and other nonkosher delicacies, like spareribs, which she lists with delight. Because of her numerous medical problems, she is restricted to eating nonspicy foods, which severely limit her enjoyment of food. Several of her children visit every night, seem

[51]

very devoted to her, and are upset about her continuing loss of weight. The nurses say that she refuses to eat in order to make her children feel guilty.

Ida Kanter. She could be called the success case of the Franklin Nursing Home. Active and well liked, she is 94 years old and was born in the United States. As a young girl she worked as a designer in the largest department store of a nearby city. Later she married and had two daughters. Her husband died years ago, and for a while she lived with a daughter. However, she found the situation too restricting, and after a short time she took her own apartment. She lived by herself for over ten years and did volunteer work. After a hospitalization, she entered Franklin. She misses her apartment but now is resigned to living here. Once she had regained her strength she became active in the nursing home. She has a no-nonsense way of evaluating what occurs in the nursing home. She recounts those things and people she does not like without bitterness and with acceptance. She notes with humor the jockeyings for power and friendship of both the residents and the staff. One particularly unpleasant woman tried to have an exclusive friendship with her, which Mrs. Kanter saw as a bid for power, and so she refused. She is similarly as perceptive and analytical about staff behaviors, many of which she dismisses as nonsense.

Jacob Strauss. Jacob Strauss, 96, has lived at Franklin for over ten years. He stays by himself, and few staff members or residents attempt to bother him because he is notoriously gruff. He entered the nursing home after the death of his wife. Staff members comment that it is not surprising that his children did not want him to live with them. He owned a store, which he turned over to a son. When he was admittted, he was fairly healthy. His primary reason for admission was loneliness, and he had trouble going to the synagogue every day. Now, however, he would be unable to live on his own. Though he uses a wheelchair, staff members are not sure whether he needs one or not.

One thing he enjoys is a card game with three other male residents. They gather at a certain time every day to play. Not much is said. He has been known to hit people who are in his way. He seems to be alert and resists any attempt to be cheered. He hears poorly but when he understands the question whether he likes the nursing home, he gives a curt no. One way that he is adept at provoking disputes among staff members is to appeal directly to the director of nurses to rectify a problem before asking a nurse on his own floor.

Principles and Strategies of Ranking: Heterogeneity and Leveling

Admission to the nursing home means that an individual was unable to muster the necessary supports to stay out of the institution. In this basic respect, all residents are the same: they are unable to function in the community. However, this equality is contradicted by the crucial fact that each resident is an individual whose separateness is continued within the nursing home. Those residents who can, struggle against the ideology of equality that institutionalization confers. The ways that residents rank one another, differentiate themselves from the others, and maintain their separateness are basic strategies of adaptation to the nursing home.

The twin dynamics of equality and differentiation reverberate throughout the institution. This point is important in matters of reciprocity and rites of passage. If prior statuses remain important and do not diminish within the nursing home over time, communitas would not be present. If individual differences are leveled over time or are perceived to be unimportant, communitas would be expected. Both leveling and individuality remain important in the nursing home; but because differences between people emerge overall more prominently than similarities, communitas has less chance of surfacing in the liminality of this rite of passage.

With acclimatization to the nursing home, residents learn to distinguish who is who: who is healthier, who is sicker, who is lucky, who is unfortunate, and so forth. Residents learn the reasons that others entered the nursing home. Though equalization occurs because all the residents are institutionalized, the individuals are marked by their former positions. Residents learn one another's family status and characterize one another accordingly. That an aloof president of a civic organization is "reduced" to entering the nursing home means to the other residents that he may not have been the model parent that he maintained himself to be, for example. Ida Kanter related an example of moral justice that seemed to correct an old wrong:

When she was a little girl, a neighbor's mother used to consider Ida's family inferior. In the neighbor's family a girl who was Ida's age displayed some of her mother's superior stance toward Ida's family. Now this girl has recently been admitted to Franklin, to Mrs. Kanter's floor, of all things. This woman is no better than the rest of them, and though she still puts on airs, she doesn't fool anyone.

[53]

On the other hand, a resident may be perceived as an unfortunate victim of an uncaring family. One resident pointed out another in this way: "This man here—his son is one of the biggest doctors in town, with a million-dollar house and a swimming pool and everything—but pop smells, so here he is." In similar ways all residents are categorized and labeled.

Importance of the Past

Retaining some of his prior affiliations and social standing, a resident may be able to maintain the status attached to past accomplishments if his present abilities allow. He may keep memberships and subscriptions current. Having the capacity to maintain outside ties of any sort is an important advantage. Some residents keep themselves detached from others in the home. Their reasons may include a reluctance to enter the nursing home, a lack of social skills, or an attempt to assert superiority. Such a resident may scoff at nursing-home activities or may refuse a series of roommates. Some residents may be misperceived as aloof, however.

Max Sager's little article in the resident's newspaper is being mentioned. It is about hearing a famous opera singer when he was a student in Berlin. "He thinks he's so much better than the rest of us," says Stanley Fierstein.

Because so many of the residents have known each other before admission, past behaviors and social standings are not erased and remain important.

Mrs. Curtin knows Leo Feldman from way back. Her husband, now deceased, used to have his shop near Leo's. "You know the way he always carries around a Yiddish newspaper? He can't read it and everyone knows it. He is just hoping to fool some people who did not know him before." Mrs. Curtin remembers that Mr. Feldman is remarkably devoted to his nice wife. But she does not quite trust him because she remembers his cutthroat business practices. He can tell such stories.

Everyone's history in this respect is important. Many of the residents have aged in a continuous "life-term social arena" (Moore 1978). They are with people in their old age whom they have known all their lives. As Moore describes the Chagga, there are both disadvantages and advantages to this experiential continuity. People in the nursing home are marked by their pasts even though they avoid talking about the past. In categorizing one another, residents rely on their knowledge of a person's education, relationship with family members (particularly the spouse), business reputation and social standing, religiosity, reputation for being honorable or not with others, and past socioeconomic, educational, commercial, or public achievements.

Priority of the Present

Residents are also classified according to their present personalities and abilities.

Gerald Wiedenbaum tries not to have anything to do with Charlie Kassin because Mr. Wiedenbaum knows that Charlie is ignorant of Jewish history, yet Charlie always wants to argue some point about it.

Boasts may be challenged:

May Festin has just been admitted, and she has been telling people that her family was always very devout and respected in the nearby town where she grew up. But Ida Kanter remembers that May's grandfather used to come to her house to eat because the Festin family did not keep kosher and Mrs. Kanter's family did.

Past achievements may be doubted or resented, as well. The fact that Max Sager used to have an artistic career is a subject sometimes raised by various staff members, but often discounted by residents, and so leveling occurs, instead.

Because present abilities overshadow past accomplishments, the significance of having "witnessed" achievement in the past is diluted and is insufficient (Myerhoff 1979). Though people may remember when a person was a college teacher, his past standing does not aid in having a relationship with him now if he is senile. His fate may seem

[55]

only more tragic. Residents make distinctions and act on them according to present circumstances. They may decide to have nothing to do with some people because they are argumentative. Knowing whether a person fights or not is an important categorizer only somewhat relevant to past behaviors.

Other Categorizers

By and large those residents who are mentally intact have minimal interaction with those who are senile. This observation agrees with that of Gubrium (1975), who described "alertness cliques" among the mentally intact residents of Murray manor, the nursing home he studied. Usually one must have some interaction and therefore some experience of a person in order to judge that he is intact. Proceeding on the assumption that someone is all right only to have consequent expectations undermined can be disturbing.

Esther Kantrowitz had an argument with Sara Meinz over the scarf Esther was wearing. The next day when Esther thought it best to make amends, Sara did not know what she was talking about.

People who have "lost their marbles," as some of the residents say, are reminders that a similar fate may await those who still have their "marbles." The mentally intact seek to avoid the impaired, but avoidance is never completely possible because confused residents can be glimpsed and heard, are present at nursing-home events, are often in elevators, at activities, or even next door, and furthermore, often wander unannounced into other residents' bedrooms. Thus, it becomes important to subdivide the category of confused residents further.

Mentally competent residents have learned that Sarah Tessler, a confused resident, is harmless, and when she wanders into one's room with her doll, she will leave satisfied if offered a piece of candy. She is treated like a child by staff members and residents alike. Everyone is fond of her, and she is like a mascot.

Another person likes to shake hands, so one shakes his hand and proceeds down the corridor. Another person who is sometimes violent is avoided consistently. Mentally intact residents would prefer that confused residents be segregated from them, but space limitations prevent such isolation. The mixing is upsetting to some:

Mr. Fierstein has been trying to persuade the social worker to change her mind about letting Mrs. Simonson remain on Mr. Fierstein's floor in the wing. "Doesn't she know that this floor is for the most able residents?" he asks rhetorically.

Residents also classify one another according to whether they were born in the United States or not. Even though most of those who are foreign born came to the United States early in the twentieth century, the distinction seems crucial. American-born residents consider themselves élite; they do not credit the European or Russian born with a real understanding of what it means to be American. The retention of old ways can be a source of ridicule:

Stanley Fierstein thinks it is terrible that Jacob Strauss continues to talk Yiddish. Isn't he in America yet? Mr. Fierstein is proud of his eighty-six years in this country and his wartime service for the United States.

Another important distinction is between males and females. There is considerable suspicion and dislike between the sexes. The men, outnumbered three to one by the women, consider them to be gossipy, man-ensnaring shrews with acid tongues. Many of the men think of themselves as a valiant minority, withstanding female advances. Many men and women prefer to have nothing to do with each other.

Mr. Abrams is talking about the women who gab and complain all the time. If only they would let him eat in peace. Mr. Abrams thinks the new round tables that have just been installed in the dining rooms to enhance conversation are fine, but the women are complaining about them already. He doesn't know why. They were upset because they weren't sitting in exactly the same places or because their rectangular trays didn't go right with the round tables. He was disgusted about the Friday night services held last week. The women want to have more to do with the actual running of the services, which he thinks is fine. Clara Cohen, that vicious woman who lives kitty-corner across from him, lit the candles and made a mess of it. Mr. Abrams was angry that the women did not put a stop to it, and if anything like that happens

[57]

again, he himself will take the candles out of her hand and order her out. He thinks it's a disgrace.

The women say the men are stupid, and they swear too much. Myerhoff (1979) writes about the female dominance exhibited at the Jewish senior center she studied. She and Gutmann (1977) have noted the many instances of powerful postmenopausal women cross-culturally. In the case of the senior center Myerhoff studied, the women's power may be related to their greater ability to exploit familial roles (1979:284). At Franklin, the power of the women seemed to have more to do with their larger numbers than with their greater control of social resources.

Separate from other measures of categorization is the boundary marker that sets apart those designated "old." As in the "poor dear" system that Hochschild (1973) described among a group of old widows, residents at Franklin at times reserve the label "old" for those most blatantly disabled or senile.

A nursing assistant is walking slowly with a small, bent-over woman. The resident is leaning heavily for support on the nursing assistant, her steps are halting and unsure, and she is muttering "buh buh buh buh buh buh" loud enough that other residents can hear her. Eddie Fink points her out to me, and says, "She's old."

At other times, however, "old" is easily applied to oneself. At the beginning of fieldwork when the social worker was introducing me to various residents and explaining that I was studying old people, responses like the following came quickly and in many cases were accompanied by laughter or a smile: "Well, you've come to the right place. We're old, all right." "I guess I could teach you a bit about that." Or even more simply: "Well, that's me!"

A crucial differentiator is between those who have children and those who do not. A person is considered blessed if he or she has children who are attentive and visit. They are élite. Childless residents watch their neighbors with children to determine whether they should be so deserving.

Sarah Zeldin is angry whenever she hears Rose complain that her daughter does not visit often enough. Why, her daughter is devoted to

Rose, and Rose ought to know it, according to Mrs. Zeldin. Mrs. Zeldin does not understand why people with children should complain at all. They are so much better off than she and other childless residents are. Mrs. Zeldin cannot really rely on anyone.

Residents who are visited by family or friends and who go out with them to restaurants or to their houses for brief stays are fortunate compared to residents who are never visited. Contact with the outside world, as represented in the visits and phone calls received, is perhaps the greatest measure of differentiation to the residents.

Residents with outside links have more resources overall. Phone calls, visits within the nursing home, and the opportunity to go out, help structure and vary time. Genuine help is available through these links, too. This fact was evident during the period of the threatened strike. Certain residents were going to stay with family members in the community during the strike while others without family were to stay in the nursing home. Some families were seen to have better resources than others and were thus superior. For example, one resident was going to have his own room in his son's house, but another was going to have to double up in his son's smaller house. Finally, residents whose local family members staunchly said they were unable to house their elderly relative had exposed the family's unwillingness to help, which under normal times was a fact that could remain hidden.

Residents with local family that exhibit the desire to help are privileged individuals. These family members can perform valuable services. They can do errands, help furnish the resident's room, and ensure that the resident's clothing is cleaned and mended properly, either by the housekeeping staff or by themselves. Those residents who are able to recruit someone to do their laundry consider themselves lucky. They do not have to worry about clothing that is lost, stolen, or mangled in the laundry service of the nursing home.

Interested family members who live nearby can protect the resident in other ways. They can and do intercede on the resident's behalf. They can talk to the social worker about a troublesome orderly or appeal to the administration regarding the fact that the resident's room is too hot or ask the nurses to try to take the resident to the bathroom more frequently. Coming from the resident, these requests carry little weight. Because family members function in the Harrison

[59]

community at large and are present or future contributors to the nursing home, they have considerable impact within the nursing home.

The family can also insulate the resident from the nursing home in certain ways. By providing home-baked favorites or specially prepared foods that the resident prefers, the institutional existence can be softened considerably. That food brought in from home can constitute a management problem for the institution does not matter much to the resident:

Frieda Kleinberg's persistent, off-and-on diarrhea has been linked to the "concoctions" that the nurses have just found out are brought in nightly by Mrs. Kleinberg's daughter. The daughter feels she is able to do something useful and meaningful for her mother; the mother loves the food. The nurses are trying to persuade the daughter to stop so her mother's medical condition can be managed better.

Family members who are nearby and willing to help can thus be effective arbiters, promulgators, and nurturers.

A separate group within the large group of residents who have children are those who have had a child die in recent years. Still others have offspring who have married Christians or who have divorced. All these distinctions enable residents to categorize one another and devise strategies for dealing with one another. Hierarchies are constructed; alliances are formed; and everyone watches everyone for changes so that new hierarchies, alliances, and strategies can be forged. Despite the leveling effects of institutionalization, therefore, Franklin residents remain separate individuals and use innovative strategies to maintain their identities in their last home.

Notebook:
Resident-Care Conference

Dr. Corning has arrived. Little by little the staff members show up. A dietician, the activities director, the physical therapist, a nursing supervisor, the director of nurses, the second-floor charge nurse, a few social workers, and I are present.

Dr. Corning starts off with what he calls a "social worker joke." It's about Mrs. Kerman, who is in the hospital. He confesses that he's always had a problem calling residents by their formal last names (as the social workers urge everyone to do): he has always called people by their first names. While he was visiting Mrs. Kerman in the hospital, her regular doctor came in to visit and called her "Mrs. Kerman." "So I'm thinking about this, wondering if I'm doing the right thing." Fran, a social worker, interjects, "I'm glad you're concerned about it." Dr. Corning continues, "So I go up to her and she's still in intensive care, and I take her hands to make contact, and I say, 'Delores, tell me, would you like me to call you Delores or Mrs. Kerman?' And she says, 'Call me Dee; it's more chummy.'" There is laughter, and there is social worker discomfort and disgruntlement rustling in the room as well.

Then Dr. Corning mentions that he's heard that Mrs. Kaufman is making a very good adjustment. She was admitted not too long ago, doesn't speak any English, has been completely blind all her life, and because her outside supports failed somehow, she had to be admitted. She was screaming and kicking in the beginning, but now she can find her way around and seems okay to him. Next, he wants to talk about how nasty some of the residents in the wing can be. There are nods around the table. Mrs. Sims, the director of nurses, says that the residents are sometimes childlike and need to be taught how to behave. Bernice, a nurse, and Pat, a dietician, add assenting comments about how difficult they can be. Dr. Corning says, "But you're the authority, right? You've got to be tough." They agree. Fran says, "I've got to take exception to your use of the word 'childlike.' That's ageism. They are not any more childlike than people on the outside, and they are not the majority of the people we have here. A lot of people here act very maturely." Lisa, another social worker, says, "I'm glad you said that." The activities director protests that sometimes the residents really do act like children. Lisa looks angry. Dr. Corning apologizes for the use of the word 'childlike.' The third social worker, Harriet, says that maybe it is fear. A nurse says maybe there should be education about how people should behave.

The subject is changed by the presentation of the first case. Harriet presents Mrs. Center, born in 1910 locally, the oldest of six children. She graduated from high school and her husband was a cobbler. They lived with her husband's parents for most of their marriage. Her husband died about ten years ago. She once had a psychotic episode, for which she was given electroshock therapy. She's always appeared depressed, isolated, and withdrawn. She was admitted to Franklin in February, after living with her brother, Mr. Strauss, with whom she argued frequently. She was diagnosed recently as schizophrenic. Though she's alert and responded correctly to the mental status exam, she has at times been on the wrong floor and hasn't known it.

Her medical problems are listed on the blackboard as follows: depression, chronic schizophrenia, arteriosclerotic heart disease, renal failure, anemia, diabetes. Eileen, a nurse, remarks about her flat affect. She brightens up somewhat when she's talked to, but mostly she sits in her room, withdrawn. She and her brother are asked to come in.

Dr. Corning talks to the brother and refers to Mrs. Center as "she" almost exclusively. She looks healthy, strong, and depressed and stares straight ahead. One of the staff members directs a question at her: "What can we do to make it better for you here?" and she responds, "Everything is all right." She adds that she does not like the food because it is unsalted. Dr. Corning wonders out loud about substituting potassium, but he is concerned about the diabetes.

Brother and sister leave. There had been many uncomfortable silences. Her birthday was yesterday, someone says. Someone else says she seems so young and strong, yet unsteady. Jean, the physical thera-

pist, says that there is a characteristic gait of depressed people that she recognized in Mrs. Center. Dr. Corning writes down that he wants to do a follow-up on Mrs. Center in three or four months.

Next to be presented is Norm Cooper, born in Russia in 1891. Lisa mentions that his birthday is in four days. He immigrated when he was 20. He had a curtain business, was married when he was 23, had two children, retired at age 65, and was always a religious man. He and his wife were admitted together a few years ago when their daughter became unable to care for them. The wife died three weeks after they were admitted. The staff feels that he dealt with the grief appropriately. His daughter and son visit frequently, but the visits are usually characterized by their sitting in silence. He gets along well with his roommate because they leave each other alone. He is fairly deaf, doesn't participate in any activities, and watches TV. He seems alert, but it's hard to tell for sure because of his deafness, and he refuses to have a hearing aid. He believes the mafia is pursuing him and sometimes becomes agitated: "It's terrible to give him a bath—unbelievable," comments Mrs. Sims, shaking her head. One of the nurses adds that it's extremely difficult to do routine tests such as blood work. She is concerned about his skin lesions, too.

He enters the room with his son. He looks old and emaciated with a round face and pendulous ears, which protrude from his head. His nose is large and prominent, and his mouth forms a taut straight line across his face. He sits down, stares ahead, and his facial expression stays like a mask. His son wears a mechanic's uniform with the word "Hank" stitched on one lapel and "Cooper Plastering Company" on the other.

Dr. Corning asks the son, "How is your father doing?" He also asks how long his father has had the hearing problem. The son replies that he thinks it's been a long time, that it is incurable, and that he's doing pretty well "for his age." He eats pretty well and seems fairly content, though "he has that persecution problem, as you know." The son says that he does all the laundry for his father because some of it would get lost in the nursing-home machines. "And his pants are always wet," adds the son.

The nurse responsible for Mr. Cooper, Mary Haggerty, looks surprised. "We think he is continent," she says. The son insists softly that every night when he visits his father, his father is wet. "He doesn't know he's doing it, you know," says the son. "It's not his fault." Mrs. Sims notes that the staff can't always tell because of certain colors. Dr.

[63]

Corning tells the son that it's important for the staff to have this information.

For the first time, Mr. Cooper is addressed directly. Dr. Corning asks him how he thinks he is doing. Mr. Cooper responds, "I'm feeling all right. I'm an old man. I'm doing okay. Everything's all right." Each one of these phrases has a long pause in between. Mr. Cooper and his son are allowed to leave.

I ask if there are some things that Mr. Cooper could be encouraged to do for himself, like bathe himself or at least be informed that bathing is important to reduce the risk of the skin lesions. Though I am told that state regulations prohibit his bathing himself, Dr. Corning thinks it's a good idea that he be told about the lesion potentiality. Mary adds that he has often been found on the back stairs, praying. He doesn't want to pray with the others. There is concern that he might get dizzy and fall down the stairs, so it is decided that he should be watched more carefully.

The meeting is about to end, but Dr. Corning brings up Mrs. Kerman again. He says that at 95 she is very alert. Long before the incident, she had specifically told him not to do anything extraordinary for her "should anything happen." Lisa asks pointedly, "And did you?" "Yes!" counters Dr. Corning adamantly. Lisa scoffs, "I don't want you to be my doctor!" The doctor says that if someone told him explicitly immediately before a procedure that he or she didn't want extraordinary measures taken, then okay. He can live with that, with not doing anything. But in this case, there was a long time lag from when Mrs. Kerman first expressed her wish for no intervention to the crisis that called for intervention. What should he do when the patient cannot express her wishes then? Deliberately using the double negative, he says that he didn't want to do nothing. Lisa says, "But you are deciding on her quality of life for her, and that's not right." When Mrs. Kerman told Dr. Corning that she wanted nothing extraordinary done, she had also explained that she'd had a long and full life and that when the time came, she wanted to go. In fact, Dr. Corning adds, she is angry at him now for what he did. But, he says, "I don't think I did the wrong thing." The nurse, Bernice, brims with disgust, "No one ever used to talk like this. In all my thirty years of nursing, there was never a question. Our job is to save lives!" She shakes her head at the social workers across the table, and walks out. The meeting is over.

[4]

Conflicting Worldviews: Home versus Hospital

The Franklin Nursing Home is a home, and it is a hospital. In some ways these concepts complement each other, and in some ways they oppose each other. Because staff members differ about their definitions of the nursing home, there is little coherence to the goals that staff members set. This lack of coherence helps prevent the formation of community and of shared rituals within the nursing home, and it creates a lonely liminality for the residents.

How we organize and perceive the world around us constitutes what social scientists call a *worldview*. The way we are brought up, schooled, and trained in our professions imparts to us particular ways of making our perceptions cohere into organized structures. We take for granted these worldviews because they are so well incorporated into our basic schemes for making sense out of stimuli. But in the sense that they are taught and learned, they are arbitrary, cultural, and not necessarily shared by others. Kept tacit, they incite conflict.

In this chapter I present some of the different worldviews on which staff members of the Franklin Nursing Home base their assumptions about their definitions of work, their goals for the residents, and their relationships with other staff members. Though the explicit philosophy of the nursing home uses a team approach to treatment goals, staff members are often at odds with one another. They rarely articulate the underlying assumptions that motivate their conflicts, and they often lapse into formulaic and stereotyped views of each other, further polarizing the splits that are due to their differing worldviews. The dichotomy between the nursing home defined as a home or as a hospital deeply pervades the motivations and actions of staff members toward residents. This split reverberates throughout the institution and is felt at all levels of resident care.[1]

Some insist that the nursing home is a home. I was talking with Tom the maintenance man about the air conditioners in the nursing home when I happened to refer to the place as an institution. Tom stiffened and said, "This is not an institution. This is a home." Those staff members who believe that Franklin should be a home also believe the nursing home should have a limited amount of control over the residents. At the same time, however, they deny how much an institutional cast holds sway over the nursing home. Gubrium notes the effort made in Murray Manor to make the nursing home look like home: "Top staff wants the Manor's public places to look like home. This means various practical things. Floor personnel are asked to wear colored uniforms instead of white ones. Nurses are discouraged from wearing caps. Music is piped onto each floor to make for a 'soothing, residential-style of living'. . . . Patients are supposed to be dressed during their waking hours, rather than remaining in hospital gowns or sleeping apparel. Holidays are celebrated on each floor 'so as to remind each and every one of them that they are still part of the world around them'" (1975:47). As a hospital, however, medical dictates take over, and control over more aspects of the residents' lives is asserted. Ambivalence and disagreement among the staff members result at times. For example, Esther Marks is obese and has hypertension. On a recent shopping trip downtown she bought smoked meats, pickled herring, and other foods of which her doctors disapprove. When she returned to the nursing home, she bragged about her purchases and announced her intention of eating them. The administrator of the home decided the foods must be confiscated. Staff members were divided about the management of this issue. A physician argued for Mrs. Marks to have her herring. Staff members are not always consistent, and the physician usually adhered to the hospital definition for his decisions, but in this case argued that she be allowed to make her own choice because this was her home. Weight was at issue in another example:

Louis Strauss has always been overweight, and attempts to control his weight since he has been a resident have barely been successful. He is angry that cakes and wine are served at parties, yet he is prohibited from having them. Family members import favorite fattening foods from home. Staff members are discussing the feasibility of enforcing his diet. He is 90 years old and has been hospitalized several times for diabetes. He has said that he does not care if he dies and has had a long and fulfilling life.

The advisability of physical restraints for some residents is often discussed according to the home-hospital dilemma:

Helen Lifton screams from the moment she is put into a geriatric chair until the moment she is taken from it. Yet, when placed in a regular chair and told to stay put, she invariably forgets, attempts to get up, and falls. She has been hospitalized for some of these falls. Her confusion becomes worse when she leaves the nursing home because of hospitalizations; however, she has not become any more accustomed to the geriatric chair and hates any kinds of restraints. Her screams disturb the other residents on the floor.

Staff discussions about such cases attempt to resolve whether to allow behavior that is "bad" for the resident or to insist on unwelcome preventive measures designed to avoid medical problems. The home-hospital dichotomy raises such issues of basic residents' rights.

Life versus Quality of Life

Of the various conceptual oppositions among the nursing home staff, the most important is between what I call *life* and *quality of life*. The two models of care implicit in them embody the home-hospital dichotomy, operate simultaneously at Franklin, and often conflict with each other. They stem from the medical model of preserving life and the social-work model of advocacy. Though Franklin was founded to provide the proper ending to aged and needy Jews, as the facility grew, it became increasingly important to render medical services to the residents. The medical model emerged as the predominant operating principle after the organization became associated with the near-by hospital, began to receive federal monies, and became affiliated with the local medical school. The nursing home thus started out as a home and evolved into a more hospital-like institution.

A considerable amount of the conflict between the social workers and the nurses is due to the fact that some of the social workers are Jewish and none of the nurses, nursing assistants, or orderlies are. It is

[67]

evident in the abhorrence displayed by many Catholic nursing personnel for any life-shortening decisions, and it contributes to misunderstanding the Jewish social workers' insistence on decisions based on
the quality of life. Staff members are at odds with each other in fulfilling the mandates of their professions. Nurses and doctors prescribe
routines to preserve life at all costs, while social workers argue for
more family and resident choice in life-preserving measures. The social workers' training socializes them to act as advocates for their
clients. When social workers help their clients manipulate social services and bureaucracies, they often view institutional management as
an obstacle. They are loathe to refer to the residents as patients.
Physicians and nurses, on the other hand, are likely to refer to residents as patients, and the nursing home is like a hospital to them.

Conflicts arise when procedures to preserve life contravene the
resident's (or family's) wishes.

*The suitability of an operation to be conducted on a terminal cancer
patient who is 87 years old was not questioned by some of the nurses,
but was considered unsuitable by social workers. The nurses and the
social workers could not understand each other's point of view in the
matter, and they criticized each other accordingly.*

The appropriateness of cardiopulmonary resuscitation (CPR) in this
setting is another case in point. While a number of the social workers
feel that CPR is unsuitable in the nursing home, many nurses consider
the questioning of CPR anathema to their morals and training to save
lives. According to one social worker, part of the conflict originates in
the different views that social workers and nursing personnel have of
physicians: "I guess nurses are taught that doctors are like gods. We
sure don't see them that way. The ones I've worked with seem so
arrogant, so sure. Often they act like they are superior to their patients. But they make mistakes. They make excuses. Nurses think the
doctors are never wrong." Nonetheless, there is also an adversarial
relationship between doctors and nurses. Nurses follow the doctors'
orders, and they must check with physicians continually about the
physical management of residents. They know how they must be
ready to fill in, take over for, and improvise for, those physicians who
are rarely there. They often resent the superiority of doctors, and they
condemn those physicians who are reluctant to visit the nursing home.
Still, they share many of the same medical values as those the physicians uphold, especially those regarding the Hippocratic oath and the

preserving of life. The discrepant points of view are irreconcilable at times.

Management of Death

Death has recently been handled by hospital routines and attitudes by and large, and home and hospital principles are at odds in this domain too. Though death looms at the residents constantly and is a subject they themselves discuss, staff members avoid the subject and cover it up whenever possible. When residents talk and joke freely about death, staff members seem repulsed. For example, Mr. Wolf said to a nursing assistant, "When I die, I'd like to be buried in Israel." The nursing assistant responded immediately, "Now, Mr. Wolf. We don't talk about dying here. We talk about living." Another example concerned a man who had not been told about a relative's death. The situation was discussed at the resident care conference:

Max Abel has been quite confused and isolated for some time. The physician asks if anything has precipitated his state. One nurse thinks he is depressed because of the death of his son-in-law, with whom he was quite close. Another nurse does not think so; she thinks he does not know about the death. No one can agree whether he knows. The nurse says to the social worker that they had been told that they weren't supposed to say anything to the resident about the death. The social worker replies that they wanted the resident to learn the news from another relative. The nurse says that she thinks no one ever told him, and her understanding was that it should be kept from him. The issue is unresolved, and no one knows whether he has the capacity to know, understand, or remember being told.

These interactions point up not only the staff's differing perceptions about the treatment of a resident but also their difficulty in sharing information among themselves.

A resident with cancer has been admitted to the nursing home from the hospital. He has been told about the diagnosis, and the staff thinks he is depressed about the news. The social worker wants the resident and the staff to "deal with" the issue of his cancer explicitly. The nurses are not sure.

[69]

When a resident is about to die, most staff members seem to withdraw. Ironically, as social and emotional supports from staff dwindle, medical props and life-prolonging interventions are fortified.[2] Nurses, nursing assistants, and orderlies sometimes discuss the impending death in hushed tones that residents are not intended to hear. When the death finally occurs, the room is closed, the physician is called so the body may be "pronounced," the next of kin is notified, the personal effects are picked up, and the body is taken away to the funeral home.

Staff time is occupied with sanitation and paperwork following the death. The chart work is finalized. Nurses' notes document the state of the resident before death; the physician or nurse writes down the time that the body was pronounced and notes the time that the family members were called, the personal belongings taken, and the body removed. The bed and room are cleaned so that a new resident may be admitted. Meanwhile, the news of the death travels quickly and stealthily among the residents, though there is little or no staff disclosure to them. Officially, silence reigns. During my fieldwork there was no memorial service; there was no notice on the bulletin boards in the hallways; there was no place to mention the event in the resident newsletter; and there was no *kaddish* (the Jewish prayer for the dead).[3] On one occasion, in protest, a resident organized a memorial service for a friend who had just died. He put up notices and was satisfied that he had expended the effort on his friend. Scoffing about the typical handling of death, he said: "When someone dies, it is as if the person never even existed. They pretend nothing has happened."

To a considerable degree, the social workers work against the conspiratorial silence that surrounds the residents regarding death. They argue for residents to be informed when someone close to them has died. They want the resident to talk about, and prepare for, his impending death. One social worker told me that she tries to listen carefully when a resident says he or she is about to die, and she attempts to be emotionally available to the person. But because there seems to be no administrative rule determining how the subject of death should be discussed and treated, each staff member approaches the subject in an individual way. In this vacuum the staff members are free to ignore or confront the subject, according to their personal tastes.

There seems to be an oscillation between the home and hospital principles in the management of death. Hospital principles were less likely to dominate fifteen years ago in a similar nursing home (Fishbein and Kaitin-Miller 1986). When a person died, everyone was told. The male residents who lived on the floor of the deceased would accompany the body as it was moved out of the nursing home. Radios and televisions were turned off during the body's exit to mark the departure. The death was noted publicly in this way. Fishbein and Kaitin-Miller do not know what created the change in policy. A social worker described her astonishment at what happens when someone dies at Franklin: "I was uncomfortable each time I saw how death was managed. All the residents are taken into the dining area and the doors are closed. Mysteriously, two men in black suits appear on the floor with a stretcher between them. They take away the body and five minutes after the residents have been taken into the dining area, they are let out again. No one ever says what just happened."

Since my fieldwork ended, Franklin may be moving away from hospital principles of managing death. There are some indications that the home recognizes that hospital principles may be detrimental. For example, it has just begun to offer an occasional memorial service. A small bulletin board labeled "In Memoriam" lists the name(s) of everyone recently deceased. If this trend continues, the nursing home will be incorporating some hospice ideas about death. The hospice movement began in reaction to the overmedicalization of death in hospitals. The principles that underlay the founding of Franklin and the national hospice movement were similar. Death was explicit in both. The differences between them have become profound, however. Overall, the nursing home attempts to prevent death for as long as possible. Hospice, on the other hand, attempts to cushion the death perceived as inevitable. In order to prepare for death and provide emotional sustenance to the dying person and his family, death is an acceptable subject of conversation. In hospice situations, personal supports are intensified until the event of death. If hospice principles are utilized again here, this nursing home will have come full circle.

Rooms and Residents

The physical layout of Franklin also reflects the home-hospital opposition. The new building is hospital-like, and the wing, which houses self-care residents, is homelike.

The residents' rooms in the wing are larger than those in most

[71]

nursing homes. Pairs of rooms share a bathroom. The doors to the corridor and to the bathrooms do not lock. Almost every room contains a television. Residents in the wing usually individualize their rooms with a few personal pieces of furniture, plants, hand-crocheted afghans, handmade lace antimacassars, photographs of offspring and other family members, civic and work-related testimonials, and, occasionally, nursery school paintings executed by the residents' great-grandchildren.

The new building is much larger and its layout more hospital-like. Most rooms are for two people. As in hospitals, a curtain between the two beds can be drawn during visits and examinations. Each room has a bathroom. Furniture is provided by the nursing home, and many have televisions and telephones. All doors to residents' rooms are labeled with the residents' names, sometimes misspelled. The rooms are minimally decorated, if at all, with residents' personal items, and the beds are usuallly covered with institutional bed linens. Hospital-like priorities dictate that nurses' stations be located centrally for maximum supervision of residents; long corridors are efficient, but limit residents' privacy. Unlocked doors ensure immediate staff intervention if necessary, but curtail resident privacy from staff and other residents.

Room Changes

Because the health status of nursing-home residents changes fairly frequently, their room placements, determined largely by level-of-care requirements, change too. A resident who is admitted following a stroke may improve after a few months of physical therapy. Conversely, a resident admitted following diabetic surgery in the hospital may have increasingly acute episodes, each requiring hospitalization. In a nursing home similar to Franklin, Rouslin made this observation:

Two residents, in particular, have suffered great hardship due to a designated change in their level of care. The first one is an 88-year-old woman, Mrs. H., who had been a resident at the [nursing home] for five years. She had been living on the fifth floor, in the same room, with the same roommate for four years. On February 2, she returned from the hospital following a bout with pneumonia. She returned as a skilled patient and, therefore, had to be moved to the second floor. On February 20, this resident went looking for her old room. She entered the room directly under her old room, pulled out a bureau drawer, the way she always had, and the drawer came flying out, as her drawer in her old room never had done. This resident fell on the floor and fractured a hip. She returned to the hospital and came back again as a skilled patient. This time she returned to yet a different room on the second floor. Meanwhile, her best friend and roommate, Mrs. M., had spent the last few weeks wandering around on the fifth floor, looking for her friend like a lost soul. She would ask staff continuously, day and night, where her friend, Mrs. H., was and spent her days wandering into other patients' rooms looking for her friend. Mrs. H.'s daughter was also very upset that her mother was not placed back on the same floor, in the same room that she was used to and complained bitterly to Administration about this. Social Service did move Mrs. H.'s roommate, Mrs. M., down to the second floor to be with her friend, Mrs. H., which meant moving the person already in that room up to the fifth floor. On February 26, both residents were moved back up to the fifth floor as Mrs. H. was no longer a skilled patient but now their old room was occupied, and they were moved into a different room. Consequently, Mrs. H.'s roommate continued going back to her old room on the fifth floor and falling asleep in her old bed. She would also put her teeth away in her old bathroom and staff would spend extra time looking for her teeth. On April 6, Mrs. H. and Mrs. M. were moved back to their original room on the fifth floor. (1981:11–12)

In addition to such typical problems, a social worker at Franklin commented how the residents become attached to their rooms: "Sometimes, when we have to make a room change, the resident (or his family) is very upset about it. It's amazing how much the particular room means to them. Sometimes they insist that it 'belongs' to them. When that happens, we have to show them the contract where it spells out how they do not own and can't claim any particular room in the nursing home." One resident spoke of her tenuous connection to her room: "Mrs. Rubin has promised me that I can keep this room, and I'd dearly like to. But I know that nothing in this world is forever, and a promise lasts only until it ends. Who knows what will happen to me, and when they will need this room? Who knows when they will decide when I should go to the 'other side' [the new building]?"

Of the 296 total residents at Franklin in 1982 (including deaths and new admissions), 31 percent required 140 separate hospitalizations of one or more days' duration, producing an average of 7 hospitalization days per resident during the year. A large proportion of these hospitalizations required a room change within the nursing home once the resident was back, and sometimes, as in the above example, more than one room change. Max Sager's year was one:

At the beginning of the year he was living in the wing. However, he became manic and was admitted to a psychiatric hospital on January 10. He was readmitted to the nursing home on February 10. Eight days later he was rehospitalized, this time in a medical facility. On March 17 he was returned to the nursing home, but his room had been changed from the first floor of the wing to the second floor of the new building. This change also entailed going from a single room to a double room. He remained in the nursing home until another psychiatric hospitalization began July 9, but in the meantime his roommate had died, and he had another roommate. He returned from the psychiatric hospital on August 16. He was depressed, withdrawn, and weak. On October 11 until November 19, he was again hospitalized at the psychiatric hospital.

Stressful room changes exacerbate the confusion of residents suffering from SDAT. Remembering where things are in one's room is a difficult task for the SDAT victim, and a room change often disrupts mastery of the room and its contents. The person may have been moved, for example, to another room on the same floor, which happens to have the location of bathroom and closet reversed from the layout of the former room. The confused resident cannot usually adapt to this kind of switch. Overall, decisions about room changes are determined by hospital-like priorities, which have been set by governmental level-of-care designations.

On the other hand, the effects of frequent moves are counterbalanced in some ways by the fact that a room in the nursing home is reserved for the resident during most hospitalizations of a few days if a new level-of-care label is not necessary. This financially expensive policy provides continuity for the residents and is a homelike consideration very unusual among nursing homes.[4]

Employees or Friends? I Only Work Here

The home-hospital dichotomy also appears in attitudes toward whether employees are friends to the residents. At times residents and staff members refer to themselves as a family.[5] This characterization is more often made by the residents in reference to the staff members than by staff members in reference to the residents.

The related idea that staff members are friends is less common. Though the friend label is used for some interactions, there are times when the unequal relationship between staff members and residents is explicitly acknowledged.

Max Sager is fond of a social worker. She is wary of his affection because she says it violates the professional distance between them, and it also seems to unnerve her personally. He has had a lithium imbalance and a history of manic-depressive illness, and she tends to utilize these concepts in order to maintain her distance. For example, she says that Mr. Sager is in his manic phase now and that is why he is more attentive to her. Today, he has walked into her office with a bottle of wine. He is happy because today marks one year since his woman friend had her stroke, and she has been recovering well. There will be a party at her house later on today, and the social worker will be transporting Mr. Sager there. To celebrate, he would like the two of them to have a glass of wine now. She refuses. He urges her to join him, but she becomes irritated. He continues to urge her, and she says that if he wants to have his wine, he may drink it in his room, but that she may not have a drink with him because she is working. She places the wine bottle directly back into his hand, gives him his cane, and tells him she will see him later. After this incident, Mr. Sager expressed his disappointment with her rigidity.

The social worker defined her role in terms of the job when she was pressed. Because Mr. Sager lives in the nursing home, he may have his glass of wine, but because she works there, she may not. This distinction served to put Mr. Sager abruptly in his place.

Many staff members act friendlike to the residents.[6] I heard of a few instances of employees inviting residents to their homes for meals or visits. Some of the experienced employees, however, say they used to do favors for the residents when asked, but now shy away from doing so, feeling trapped by the pattern. They advised me to be wary, explaining that residents always escalate their first reasonable wishes into unremitting demands for increased help, involvement, and errands.

When the strike threatened, many residents who had believed that the nursing assistants, orderlies, and other union employees were their friends had their understanding abruptly clarified. As bystanders and direct victims of the administration-union dispute, the residents had to recognize organizational differences and their effects. The residents were ideologically torn during the negotiations, for many have prounion sentiments, which they attempted to maintain. Yet, their commitment to union solidarity and ideas of friendship was insulted by the employees' seeming willingness to sacrifice resident care to their own interests. Because many residents recognized this discrepancy, they accurately understood their basic isolation. The threat of strike made the lines clear.

Rehabilitation versus Maintenance

The physical therapy room at Franklin is the one place where residents seem free to talk, express fear and hope, and air complaints. Significantly, the physical therapist is emotionally involved with the residents and cares about them. She also intervenes in their defense when she feels it is necessary.

She is telling me about the time one of the residents came to physical therapy and had a bruise that, to the physical therapist, looked suspicious. She was sticking her neck out, she knew, by reporting it, but she decided to act. She phoned the charge nurse on the resident's floor and reported it. She also wrote it up. Though she knew she was inviting employee resentment and anger by her actions, she felt it was important to be a resident's advocate and agent for change in this way. She was letting employees on the floor know that she was not going to avoid difficult issues and help cover things up.

The physical therapy room seems a place apart within the nursing home. A different atmosphere is apparent there as residents share stories, make jokes, smile, laugh, and flirt with each other. They also work hard. Many of them struggle with pain to undergo exercise routines.

The physical therapist says that the residents know they can talk about anything they want in this safe room. Crediting herself, she says that she is on their side, that she will act on their behalf, and that she will not betray their confidences. The personal investment she makes in her work is evident in several ways. Her assistants appear, like her,

[76]

genuinely to like the residents. They show interest in the stories that the residents relate. Sexual humor, courtship stories, and future potential prospects are frequent subjects that residents and staff members alike enjoy. Progress is made in this room. Residents are encouraged, supported, and pushed to work harder, not to give up, to try again. Encouragement to live and struggle is fostered in this room. Each resident's effort to improve physical functioning serves as a model for active behavior elsewhere, underscoring the basic message of the physical therapy room: residents should try, should continue to strive.

In the physical therapy room residents have the opportunity to be themselves at the same time that they assert their commonality. The ease with which they talk with each other and with the physical therapy staff about their pasts as well as about what is currently happening in their lives confers a special aura to the room and the hard work that goes on within it. Physical therapy is frustrating, painful, and arduous; results can take a long time to materialize. Residents make strides, sometimes only to relapse. But residents who come to physical therapy are encouraged to continue to work against the pain and the odds of failure, and they often have astonishing results. Murphy, an anthropologist who is quadraplegic, describes his physical therapy:

The leg exercises became at once longer and less exhausting. Even though I pushed back harder than before, the therapist seemed chronically dissatisfied with my performance—urging, cajoling, and nagging me onward until I would just give up and stop. I soon discovered that this was standard procedure, part of a game played by therapist, patient, and often, an audience. One day, for example, a young paraplegic woman was helped to her feet, given a walker, and told to walk. After about five steps, she told the therapist, who was walking just behind her, that she was tired and wanted to stop. The therapist told her that she was giving up too soon and ordered her to continue. The other therapists and their patients echoed him, telling her that she could do it, forming a cheering section as she struggled onward. She soon stopped again, this time begging to be put back in the wheelchair, but the therapist was adamant. Finally, after she broke down in tears and showed signs of collapsing, the chair was brought up behind her and she fell into it. Everybody in the gym applauded, and she wiped away the tears and grinned in triumph. The patients soon get into the spirit of the game, knowing that today's painful overreach may become tomorrow's

[77]

routine accomplishment. Some even see it as a way of defying their doctors, who tend toward quite conservative prognoses. . . . There is some danger that doctors' predictions can also induce despair, and the exhortations of the therapists are meant to counteract the sometimes overpowering urge to give up. (1987:50–51)

This extraordinary passage describes the immense feelings of helplessness and gloom coupled with the kinds of victories that can be experienced through the work of physical therapy. I suggest that in the physical therapy room, two important processes are at work that rarely surface otherwise in the nursing home: residents interact meaningfully with each other and with the staff members through talk, jokes, reminiscences, complaints, and so forth; and they struggle and work with progress as their almost impossible goal. Here are the ingredients for community building and ritual formation. Regardless of the variety of the personalities struggling together, the residents share anguish and success. And in this room, nothing is handed to them gratis. Everything that they accomplish they have earned by hard work. They reciprocate and act as tough adults—with obstacles and with dreams.

There is the opposing thread, however. As frailer people are admitted, rehabilitation seems to be an increasingly less relevant goal of the nursing home. When the physical therapist asks nurses which residents could use physical therapy, they offer few, if any, names. When the physical therapist persists in asking or checks among the residents herself, she finds suitable candidates. When she identifies them to the nurses, they normally consent, but they do not always cooperate in arranging for them to be transported to and from the physical therapy room, nor do they cooperate in minimal follow-up care.

A stroke patient who had no use of his legs upon admission attended physical therapy three times a week. After prodding by the physical therapy staff, the resident was walking with the aid of a walker. However, back on the fourth floor, where his room was, the nursing staff did nothing to supplement the gains that had been made in the physical therapy sessions. While there are standing orders for nursing assistants and orderlies throughout the institution to do range of motion exercises (simple exercises to stimulate muscles in arms and legs in order to improve strength and mobility) with all the residents, they are rarely done. The routine of the institution takes a higher priority.

[78]

Therefore, nails are cleaned, hair is brushed, and beds are made while residents remain sitting in chairs, watching. Staff members do their jobs; the residents wait.

The effort to rehabilitate residents competes with the opposing notion that maintenance of residents at their current level of functioning is adequate. Passivity often dominates.

The home-hospital split within this nursing home is profound and affects many aspects of resident care. Adherence to one worldview or the other prevents the smooth teamwork operation that most staff members say they desire.

Notebook:
Physical Therapy

*I arrive at the physical therapy (PT) room at 9:30 A.M. Helen Safrin
has her legs up and has hot packs on one knee. She calls the PT room
Pain and Torture. She also says she comes to socialize.*

*Mr. Abrams from the second floor is walking between two parallel
bars. He's calling Mrs. Safrin "darling" and "sweetheart." She says,
"Are you talking to me?" He tells her he'd like her to take her blouse
off. She fires back, "Oh Mr. Abrams, I didn't know we were so close."
I see Gerald Wiedenbaum's wife is here. She is severely demented.
Mr. Wiedenbaum says she doesn't recognize him anymore. However,
she looks as if she understands what someone is saying to her, and she
is answering correctly right now.*

*Jean Connolly, the physical therapist in charge, calls me over to
meet Mary Gottschalk. As Jean holds Mrs. Gottschalk's arm and
hand, Mrs. Gottschalk relates how she used to walk and do everything
for herself when she was first admitted. Then her muscles degenerated
and she had surgery, which alleviated pain but worsened her mobility. She makes slow progress in physical therapy. Mrs. Gottschalk
lives on the fourth floor. "It's bad up there," she says. Jean concurs.
Sometimes, residents are sent to physical therapy improperly washed,
and Jean has to send them back. Jean has seen staff members on the
fourth floor do nothing when someone is screaming. "It's murder to
chart up there. The aides and everybody are talking so much, it's so
noisy. You go crazy trying to chart." Mrs. Gottschalk says how nice it
is in the PT room.*

*Jean has greeted Herm Silver. He's singing songs and making pep-
pery remarks. "You don't mind if I breathe, do ya?" he challenges*

Jean, and she retorts, "We're going to get along today, aren't we?" Off and on, he commands attention as his voice rises in song. Jean's assistants, Helena and Ellen, do range-of-motion exercises, and they walk the residents when possible. One of them is doing range-of-motion exercises on Herm while he sings and makes remarks.

Jean tells me about Herb Rosenzweig, who was a great success in physical therapy. He was so contorted that he could barely move, and he couldn't walk at all. His drive was amazing, and he progressed very fast. He was determined to walk, and he continued to improve. But then he got a bad cold and was set back. He continued to work and improve. Then he became sick again, and now has pneumonia and is in the hospital. She called him there, and he was delighted to hear from her.

A man is wheeled into the room and Jean says to me, "Watch this: Hello Joseph!" she calls out very loudly and very cheerfully. "How're ya doing? Good?" Her face is close to his, and he smiles and answers her with some animation. She says to me, "He doesn't respond at all on his floor. They don't believe that I get this much out of him down here."

Most of their work is maintenance rather than real rehabilitation, though at times residents make great strides. She attributes most of the progress to the residents' work. When she first came here two years ago, there were many residents whom the staff assumed couldn't walk at all. The staff on the floors made little effort to identify those who could make improvements. Jean now thinks she has identified most of them, but she still meets with nurse resistance. "It's an uphill battle," sighs Jean, "because we work with a person down here in the PT room maybe three or five times a week, but when they go back to the floors, they just sit, and the nursing assistants and nurses don't walk them or do the range-of-motion exercises with them like they're supposed to. It's frustrating."

Jean now tells me about Utka Markoff. She is a new resident, a stroke victim. Jean is proud of her, though Mrs. Markoff has been timid and fearful about improving. Every day she tells Jean, Helena, and Ellen of her aches and pains, and she cries when they urge her on. Businesslike, they tell her that they don't want to hear the complaints. They want to get right to work and see how far she can walk this time. The other day she managed to walk all the way down the corridor with one person on each side of her, cajoling and praising her the whole time. Jean got all the people in the occupational therapy room to come out and praise her too, and there is a sign in the PT room stating how many steps Utka took. Mrs. Markoff was overjoyed when she accomplished the walk.

On the floors upstairs it's different, explains Jean. There, the patient-to-staff ratio is 7:1 and here it is 1:1. There they don't stay interested in the patient. Monday mornings in PT are especially pathetic because the residents have gone backwards over the weekend because the weekend staff does no range-of-motion exercises or walking of the residents at all. There is always much ground to be made up.

Now Jean is working on Doris Moerman. Jean is telling me about Mrs. Moerman as she works, and Mrs. Moerman is smiling, nodding. She had a stroke and was doing very well with physical therapy. Then ("there is no justice," says Jean), she had another stroke, and this stroke, Jean whispers, was worse and affected her mind. She was a superintelligent lady, good dresser, worked in Washington. It's not fair. Now, Jean urges Doris to stand up and places her hands around the handles of the walker. "Pick up the walker, Doris. Stand up straighter. I'm doing all the work, Doris. Come on. Now don't walk like an old lady, Doris! Pick up the walker. That's better. Come on." Doris grins with the praise, but I can see that she is doing very little for herself. Jean is urging, sometimes brusquely, always warmly.

Herm Silver is coming down the hall, escorted by both Helena and Ellen; first he's singing an Irish shanty and now he's pretending to be Chinese. Then he says to me, "If you don't stop that, I'll hit you." Jean tells him to behave himself. He resumes a more good-natured tack. Jean tells me in such a way that he can hear that he is a famous spoon collector. There was an article in the newspaper about him. "Right, Herm?" He grins and nods. Now he's singing, "Your eyes are still blue, because I'm a Jew. . . ."

Jean and I go over to Esther Sahlins and sit down. When Esther came here about two years ago ("right, Esther?") she walked all over the building, up and down. Then she had a stroke, which left her unable to walk. She was so wobbly it scared Jean every time they got her up to practice. Now Jean asks her to tell me about her boyfriend, Johnnie. Esther laughs and says that every night she takes her boyfriend Johnnie to bed with her. She's famous for this joke. When someone whom she'd told about Johnnie for a long time came to visit and wanted to meet Johnnie, Esther had to say, "Oh, he just left" because, she explained to me, Johnnie is the hospital gown, and she had just taken it off. Jean says, "Esther, tell us about your marriage."

[82]

Esther tells how she lived on the third floor, and new people moved into the second floor. One day she couldn't get into her apartment, and the young man from the second floor helped her get in. They got married ten days later. He was very handsome. He worked in a manual trade that excluded Jews, so he wore a cross on his forehead and "passed." "And tell about the gambling, Esther," urges Jean. He loved to gamble and would shoot craps in the backyard. One day he made seventeen hundred dollars, and he came over to Esther's and said, "C'mon, we're going out, get dressed." "So, I got all dolled up, and he came in his overalls." She laughs at the memory. They were married for fifty years. "No one thought it would last," chuckles Esther.

"It was too bad he had to die so quick," she remembers. Jean says, "But you had such a long time together. Fifty years." Esther persists and says, "But the way it happened—so quick. He was at the doctor's office when it happened, a heart attack, I guess." Now we are up, and Esther is walking with the walker, but going too fast, worrying Jean. Esther tells Jean that she needed to go to the bathroom yesterday, and she rang for help, but it was taking too long for the nursing assistant to come, so she went to the bathroom alone. "Oh, no," groans Jean, "you shouldn't do that." We're walking in the corridor now, and someone who passes says, "How're you doing, Esther?" and she answers lightly, "I'm going to have a baby." Then she says to us, "If my husband could see me now, he'd be buried again. I used to have blond hair."

Utka Markoff is going to try to walk now. Jean takes one arm and helps Mrs. Markoff put her weight on the walker. Mrs. Markoff's brother is watching and praising from behind her. Mrs. Markoff is whimpering softly, saying that she can't do it, but Jean won't hear of it. Dr. Corning comes by and watches, and Mrs. Markoff seems buoyed up by his being in the audience. She has trouble getting one foot out straight in front of her so that she can put weight on it. Jean almost scolds her to get it straight. It twists up. Jean asks Helena to get another walker that might be a better size. They try that. Still, it's slow going, and it's hard. We get almost to the end of the corridor, but Mrs. Markoff can't go any further, and Jean lets her stop. "Well, Utka, you were trying, but it wasn't good today, I have to tell you that. So we'll stop now, but you have to come back down this afternoon because it wasn't good." "Thank you, Jean," answers Mrs. Markoff, "you are a good teacher."

There are two other women: one who has been here many years, "a

[83]

screamer who they thought couldn't walk, but who walks now," and one with Parkinson's "who has the most beautiful smile if you can get her to smile." Jean tries and tries, but finally concludes that the woman with Parkinson's is too medicated today. She doesn't blame the staff upstairs. "This woman also does a lot of screaming, and it's impossible to listen to someone screaming and screaming for too long. It's too hard on the other residents."

I meet Josephine Gustafson, who has been here three months and whose son is a resident in the wing. She has six great-grandchildren, the youngest two weeks old. He was brought in to meet his great-grandmother yesterday. Her eyes sparkle as she tells about it. She's articulate though her false teeth are loose and go up and down as she talks.

Jean sees eighty-four residents a week. The therapy of some could probably be discontinued, but she'd hate to do it to them. "It's common sense," she says "to want people to do better than they're doing. It's good to teach them how to do things for themselves, like button their clothes, put on their shoes, and things like that. And you'd think that it would make the nurses' work easier if the residents could do more for themselves. But the nurses seem to prefer to do things for the residents. It's easier for them, somehow, but I disagree with that approach."

"It's hard here," she continues. "Staff members need to work together here more, but they don't. People seem to do the minimum; they say they're 'not aware' of problems, and so forth. It's unprofessional, terrible. You should do the best you can."

We go to lunch, and Helena and Ellen join us. Helena has been working here only five months, but her help has made Jean's life much easier. Jean couldn't go on vacation before. What would happen to the residents while she was gone? She knows she shouldn't be so involved, but she is. For a while she had another assistant who didn't work out because she brought all her personal problems to work and told the residents about them. Though the residents listened politely and didn't seem to mind, some of them told Jean that they didn't like her disclosures. Jean thinks it's not right. "These people are too dignified to hear this stuff; they're offended by it." Jean let her go.

Helena calls the PT room a "neutral zone" of joking and socializing, with Jean, Ellen, and Helena the audience. They also act as mediators and expediters for the resident. Jean just called the nurse to report a rash even though the call annoyed the nurse. "I don't care if it bugs them; I'll do it anyhow."

"It's the same thing at all nursing homes," she says, "but for what they're paying here, they ought to be treated like kings and queens. Everything should revolve around the resident, but you know it doesn't. The nurses come first here, and I say it should be the resident who comes first."

Notebook:
The Threatened Strike

9:15 A.M. *Today it will be decided whether there will be a strike. I learn that labor and management are meeting now. Bernice says the strike stirs up her own feelings, feelings of things not being fair to people like her. She's a management nurse, directly under the director of nurses. Therefore she can't strike, but she is not considered a department head. So when things go well, she's not given any particular recognition. The tension is a terrible strain on her. No one's talking, everyone has gripes, it's really awful. Did I know that she's going to be retiring soon and moving away?*

It rankles her that she has to hear news of the strike from Betty, the spokesperson for the union, who is technically below her. The poor patients, she says. Those poor things, packing up their bags, and they have so few things, and those things are so precious. She still can't get over how sad it is when one of them dies and she has to pack up their things: there is so little left, maybe one suitcase full. You have to wonder, she tells me, what it's all about in between—you start out with nothing and you end up with so little—what's the rat race in between all about? She finishes photocopying the list of nurses and others who will be on duty if there is a strike, and she heads down the hall.

I go into the front lobby. Charlie Kassin is there, smoking a cigarette. He thinks there is too much fuss, but believes that the "workermen" should get raises. He remembers a strike in 1938 and how he was an independent and was let through the lines. He's been busy packing up his room all morning. He'll stay with one of his daughters, though he hasn't decided which one. What do the other residents think about the strike, I ask. "They're old," he answers. "What do they care?"

A man comes by whom I haven't met and we introduce ourselves. He hits his chest and says, "Rosen, Jew." He's on the fourth floor, and all he cares about is that he should get his meals. Mr. Kassin says the cook will be gone too, you know. "So?" counters Mr. Rosen. "I should walk out and get myself something to eat, no big deal." He shrugs his shoulders simply. His daughters live nearby, and he'll manage if he needs something.

I find Mrs. Sims in her office, and she waves me in. She talks very fast and reels off the strike preparations. She shows me lists of things and rummages through the papers she's preparing. She lights a cigarette. All the RNs are on duty. Lots of volunteers from the community have been lined up. People from the nursing pools have signed up. Obtaining this commitment was hard because the nursing home didn't know if the pools would come through the line or not. Special stickers have been prepared for all residents indicating who needs what, whether the person is incontinent, whether he or she chokes on food, whether he or she is diabetic, whether he or she is combative. It's hard to "tag" people, however. They've put wristbands on everyone, but the bands do not stay on because the residents work and work at them until they come off. "Jewish people don't like to be tagged; they have this fear of it. A lot of our residents came out of the Holocaust, and they're afraid of being tagged. That's why we're going to do stickers, instead."

They've abolished the supervisory positions for the strike, so that all heads of departments will be on the floors. They've prepared briefs on each resident, which include information on the resident's routine, the important information listed on the stickers, information about dressings, and so forth.

The wing will be closed down so there will be only four floors to contend with. Residents with no relatives will be moved into the new building. Friends will be put together if possible. The moves are traumatic, and many of the residents are confused. All have their things packed.

Mrs. Sims is particularly concerned about falls. It's important to maintain resident routines; for example, residents are used to having their shoes put in just the right place, and if they're not there, the resident can trip over them and fall. Residents who are going home

[87]

with families are worried about whether their rooms will be here when they come back.

Food will be bulk rather than on individual trays. It will be modified so that diabetics and those on salt-free diets will be able to eat it. Those who are incontinent will be wearing diapers all the time because there won't be enough staff members to get people to the bathrooms often enough. Residents who cannot dress themselves will be in johnnies and robes. The tension is very high, comments Mrs. Sims. She doesn't think people in such a place should strike. There should be binding arbitration instead. She predicts that many of the families won't be able to handle the residents they take home, and that after a day or so the families will be bringing them back. There's also a deep relationship between the resident and the nursing assistant which is threatened because of the strike. Residents don't understand.

The medical director will be here during the strike, and ambulances will come through the line. All supplies have been prepurchased. There will be security in the yard for those who want to cross the picket line. There will be a pick-up point for workers who park away from the facility to avoid vandalization of their cars. Staff members have been very cooperative. Each staff member who comes in will be working twelve-hour shifts. One nurse is coming with her baby, whom she will breast-feed on the job. Social service personnel have been working especially hard, counseling families and consoling residents.

There will be no recreational activities, though the volunteers will try to involve the residents during the time. Mrs. Sims thinks the union demands are fairly legitimate, but money is a real problem. Most residents are on Medicaid, which is paid by the state, and you can't get around that. Shortfalls in the budget are made up for by the community, but do not eliminate the deficit.

What else? Staff will man the laundry: all dishes will be paper plates. Unfortunately, the hospitals will take only the sickest patients. The others will be treated as maintenance patients even though they're sick. Some secretaries will be coming in; they have told her they're worried about how they'll react to working with the residents. Will they throw up when they do work on their bodies, for example?

Mrs. Sims has more preparations to make, so I leave her office. I go to another nursing supervisor, Madeleine. She laughs when I ask her what she thinks about the strike and asks if I'm going to write about this for the newpaper or something. I remind her about my policy of changing people's names and protecting confidentiality. She thinks the strike is not going to happen. But it's so much work to prepare just in case. She thinks the staff should be paid more, but she doesn't think they should strike. Behind Madeleine are stacks of papers, each page representing the important information on each resident. She laments the tension of these preparations. It's assumed that all non-union people will work twelve-hour shifts, but that's a hardship on some, she reminds me. She knows a few people who were scheduled to go away for vacation. Someone else had a wedding to go to and she's supposed to drop it.

While we're talking one of the social workers joins us. She has heard it was looking more positive, but Madeleine relates more ominous information. They talk about where to park should there be a strike. Bess comes into the office with her suitcase. She will stay here so she won't have to cross picket lines. Madeleine is angry that the nursing home has no insurance to cover damage to employee property, and yet the nursing home expects the staff to come in anyhow. The labor lawyer explained yesterday that anyone wishing to work is to wait in front of the line until a policeman escorts him or her inside. Madeleine says that she heard one of the nursing assistants say that she doesn't mind going on strike because she'll be glad not to do the toilets for a while.

After I leave, I see Fran hurrying down the hall with her usual cup of coffee. She also talks about the tension. One thing she has learned is that some families are fantastically great, and others are awful. Some of the families have given weak excuses for not taking their relatives home. Some who have promised to take their elderly relative home have changed their minds. Franklin has to insist because now the rooms have been promised to others.

Now I go up to the second floor. I see Mrs. Herman in her wheel-chair and her private duty nurse, Dolly. I ask Dolly if she's going to be affected even though she's privately hired. No, she isn't, but she's concerned about the mechanics of getting in and out, and she thinks she'll have to arrange to get some sort of pass. In saying hello to Mrs. Herman, I say what a beautiful day it is outside, and she answers me by saying that it is not a beautiful day inside. Mrs. Herman says that the strike is a terrible thing. Dolly looks surprised that Mrs. Herman has an opinion. Max Sager comes by and when I ask him what he thinks about the strike, he says, "What am I going to do? Move to Scotland?" Mr. Sager excuses himself, and I talk to Julio, one of the orderlies on the floor. He says that the proposed raise is nothing *considering inflation over three years. They want to take away lunch or extend the shift to 3:30. And they want you to call in three hours before your shift starts to give them notice if you're sick. "That's crazy," he says. You'd have to wake up at 4:00 A.M. to see if you are sick, and then call in. The phone at the nurses' station rings; it's Betty relating that there will be another meeting in a few minutes.*

Some of the residents are getting ready to go to the zoo. The wheelchairs are lined up near the elevator.

I go to see Mrs. Zeldin in the wing. She is upset and says that she is in the way. Other people have families to go to, but they are also upset and do not want to leave. Everyone has suitcases on their beds, she tells me. Everyone's worried about family members being too busy for them. She's worried that if she goes to the "other side" she will end up there. It upsets her to witness some of the people there, people who are really sick. They cry out in the night. And she can't get any news. No one tells her anything. She found out from someone that there is to be a meeting, but otherwise, why don't they tell her what's going on? People's bags are on their beds, their fans and TVs are packed, their telephones are being unplugged. She won't even know her telephone number if she has to move. How could she choose which things to take? Why bother to pack? Everything is precious, and she couldn't pack it all. "Look," she gestures to me, "here's my stationery and stamps all set out the way I like it. Where will it be in another room?" What about poor Mrs. Freed, across from Mrs. Zeldin, who sometimes wets herself. Who's going to change her? What about Mrs. Zeldin's niece, who might visit during the strike? How will she get through? She thinks that the staff should get a raise, but on the other hand, she sees that they do not work very hard. She's glad I came right now so that she could unload. She says, "Institutionalized people get accustomed to the way things are inside, and they get afraid to go out." I tell Mrs. Zeldin that I will call her during the strike. She refers to the commotion that the threatened strike is causing as the "eruption and the corruption." When I leave we hold up our crossed fingers.

At 2:00 P.M., the negotiation deadline, I check if there's word about the strike. The time has been extended, and both sides are still talking. From home, at 4:45 P.M., I call Franklin and am told that the strike has been averted.

[5]

The Total Institution

Researchers such as Gubrium (1975) and Retsinas (1986) have noted discrepancies between the nursing homes they studied and the Goffman (1961) prototype of the "total institution." My purpose in teasing out similarities and differences is not just to distinguish the Franklin Nursing Home from the classic total institution but to clarify the limitations of Goffman's model and to proceed beyond it toward a more revealing understanding of how nursing home life is a ritual-less rite of passage.

Bureaucracy

In the Franklin Nursing Home, a bureaucracy with separate departments and differentially defined jobs, the hierarchies, channels, and routines largely determine how the nursing home work is defined and done. Weber (1947) likened bureaucracies to giant machines in which individuals are cogs, subordinated to the smooth functioning of the machine. Weber noted how bureaucratic harmony constrained the earlier American values of frontier individuality and adventurousness. As Bensman and Vidich put it: "Bureaucracy implies—at least at the level of work—a series of external, objective, legalistic constraints which make each individual surrender—for the sake of the organization and his personal success within it—his own autonomy, his own rhythm of work, and his own ability and desire to define goals for himself and to execute them on an individual basis" (1971:25–26). Each level of hierarchical relations within the organization has a specifically defined sphere of jurisdiction and is organized according to rationally determined procedures, goals, and means for securing ends. Staffing is dictated by priorities such as vacation time and budget constraints. Staff members interact with residents in terms of their jobs and because of organizational exigency. Thus, nurses, nursing assistants, orderlies, social workers, housekeepers, kitchen workers, and administrators in the nursing home usually do not have time to talk with residents because their bureaucratically defined work consists of other activities, such as completing forms, dispensing medications, making beds, and performing various duties consistent with their job descriptions. These priorities also result in the noncontinuity of resident care because it matters less who does the job than that the job is done.

The Union

Union rules and the threat of strike exert considerable control over how the nursing home is managed.[1] Rules are followed narrowly and minimally, and job performance is linked directly to union-defined guidelines. Relationships between union employees—nurses, nursing assistants, orderlies, kitchen and housekeeping staffs—and administrative staff are often perceived as adversarial, and disputes center on bureaucratic interpretations of the rules. Jobs are often carried out in discretely defined segments. "That's not my job" or "I am not your aide" or "Your orderly is on his break" are commonly given reasons for defining the limitations of one's responsibility to the residents. Many of the residents know this reality:

Esther Sahlins has been discussing the possibility of a strike. Though she is fond of several of the housekeeping employees whom she knows, she is aware of how little pride they invest in their jobs. "When Elsie comes in my room to clean, she just 'tickles' the dust under my bed. She's not bothering herself much. Maybe they should get more pay, though."

When to give baths, when to take breaks, whether to take a resident to the bathroom when he requests it are decisions linked to the employee's interpretation of the job.

The threatened strike exposed bureaucratic principles underlying the operation of the nursing home. It created separate sets of tensions in each department. Department heads vied with the employees below them. Lines of authority and hierarchy, though always tacitly present, were conspicuous when the strike was an ominous possibility.

Hierarchy and Territory

Several implicit hierarchies—medical, administrative, nursing, and social service—operate within the bureaucracy, sometimes in conflict. Ostensibly, the physician is in charge of the resident's care—of the resident's medical status, of his medications, of changes in his diet, of restrictions in behaviors. But it is the nurses, the nursing assistants, and the orderlies who deliver the orders, who institute and administer the care. They differentially interpret the orders that have been issued.

The administration (administrative director, assistant administrator and staff, and departmental heads) constitute management, while those below them in each hierarchy are unionized. The administrator is the head of the institution, but he is also a liaison person to the community. He must satisfy the board of trustees; he attempts to please residents and their families; he does program and financial planning; he oversees the staff; and he deals with the administration of the neighboring hospital.

The nursing hierarchy is headed by the director of nurses, who determines schedules and juggles the conflict between adequate staffing and cost containment.

Today one LPN and one nursing assistant on the second floor have called in sick. Mrs. Sims, the director of nurses, determines that because two of the residents on that floor are in the hospital, the management of the floor will not be hurt by the loss of two staff members during the shift. This judgment collides, however, with that of the charge nurse on the floor, who feels that her shift has been understaffed already and cannot bear the extra patient load. She is determining how the dressings will be changed and how the showers will be supervised. Mrs. Sims, on the other hand, as part of administration, is determining staffing numbers partially on the basis of the budget. Though she may call up a nurse from the pool, they must be

[93]

paid more than her regular staff. Mrs. Sims is therefore reluctant to use the pool and decides to understaff today instead.

This frequent problem originates in conflicting pressures, on the one hand, to keep costs contained and, on the other hand, to provide adequate care.

Nursing assistants and orderlies have the most contact with residents. Licensed practical nurses have more contact with residents than do registered nurses, who spend much of their time in state-required paperwork and the planning of staffing for the floor. Each separate nursing shift is operated like a small fiefdom with the charge nurse as boss. Each charge nurse interprets the notes and orders from the physician and other staff members. Within the limits set down by the physician, she determines how to handle the residents. Because the procedures and principles change with a new charge nurse on each shift, inconsistencies and conflicts in patient care result.

The charge nurse on the day shift on the fourth floor has determined that Mrs. Simon will wear absorbent pads during her shift because of her tendency to be incontinent. The charge nurse on the evening shift thinks that residents should not wear absorbent pads, if possible, and she makes sure that her staff take Mrs. Simon to the bathroom frequently enough to control the incontinence. Social workers' attempts to influence the day charge nurse to adopt the same policy as the evening nurse meet with an offronted, territorial response. Her shift is harder, she maintains, because there are more activities taking place, and her staff is busier with other tasks.

Charge nurses choose the specific procedures regarding the treatment of bedsores, taking residents to activities, taking residents for walks, determining the appropriateness of certain medications, and managing incontinence, among other things. Though the senior nurses in administration considered the problem of abrupt changes in resident-care policies from shift to shift (as many as three per twenty-four-hour period) to be serious, no solution was found during the period of fieldwork. Sovereignty over one's particular shift remained in force.

The social service department constitutes another separate hierarchy within the nursing home. Social workers often conflict directly with the nursing hierarchy.

A resident made a request to a social worker about a change in diet. The social worker talked directly to the physician. The nurse expected that the resident would make such a request to her rather than to the social worker, and she was angry at the social worker for not referring the request to her. Meanwhile, the dietician had received the changed order from the physician. She was annoyed because the resident had told her that the food was fine. She expected dietary changes to come through the nursing and physician hierarchies rather than through the social-worker hierarchy. Because this request was channeled through social service, she felt that her job of working out minor changes in diet and food preferences directly with the resident and the nursing staff had been undermined; the change became an order from the physician via the social service department and seemed to imply that she had resisted the resident's wishes.

Family members often direct complaints to the social worker rather than to specific care givers, such as the nursing assistant, orderly, or nurse. Social workers are supposed to solve various problems: they track down missing clothing from the laundry; they arrange shopping trips for residents or do the errands themselves; they effect changes in diet; they deal with roommate problems and room changes; they intercede between family members and the resident; and generally they try to alleviate social and personal problems.

Conflicts between the nurses and the social workers arise because of overlap in responsibilities and in territory, as well as from their different points of view. When the social worker suggests to a nurse, an aide, or an orderly that the resident should be addressed by formal surname, a disdainful reaction often results. The social worker seems to have intruded into their work. In doing their work, social workers frequently offer suggestions or make requests of other staff members. Nurses, nursing assistants, and orderlies react as if they have been criticized. They often say that social workers do not know what it is like to care for sick, often demented, often combative, needy individuals on a continual basis. Because the hierarchies and worldviews of social workers and nurses are parallel and distinct, this observation is valid. Unlike the nursing assistants and orderlies, the social workers do not give primary, physical care to the residents. They do not feed, walk, lift, or bathe the residents, nor do most of them want to. Meanwhile, the social workers say that their suggestions are not taken

[95]

seriously and that other staff members are ignorant of their work. They know they are seen as troublemakers. At other times, however, nurses, nursing assistants, and orderlies seem to expect too much from the social worker. The social worker should be able to solve the roommate problem or the family problem or the whining problem. These problems make the work of the nursing assistants, orderlies, and nurses more difficult, and they should be fixed magically by the social workers. Misunderstandings naturally abound.

One of the social workers attempted to teach nursing assistants and orderlies exactly what it is that social workers do in order to try to bridge this gap. She was surprised that the nursing assistants and orderlies assumed that residents merely walked into the institution to be admitted. They had no awareness of the admission procedures that social workers administer and less understanding of the social workers' roles than she had expected.

Social workers blame the administration for not supporting them. At times they are intimidated by the resentment they know they incur. Each group says defensively that the other group does not understand the difficulty and complexity of its work, and each group is right.

The Total Institution

Goffman's description of total institutions elucidated characteristics that unite distinct institutional organizations.[2] The papers collected in his book *Asylums* (1961), based mainly on his study of a mental hospital, detailed these characteristics, described the "career" or passage of inmates through the institution, portrayed the staff world and the inmate world, and itemized the points of contact between inmates and staff.[3] As in his *Presentation of the Self in Everyday Life* (1959), Goffman was interested not only in how the total institution operated—its raison d'être and its structure—but also how the individual inmate negotiated his way through the system, presenting and preserving his self in the face of institutional onslaught. As he stated: "Sociologists have always had a vested interest in pointing to the ways in which the individual is formed by groups, identifies with groups, and wilts away unless he obtains emotional support from groups. But when we closely observe what goes on in a social role, a spate of sociable interaction, a social establishment—or in any other unit of social organization—embracement of the unit is not all that we see. We always find the individual employing methods to keep some distance, some elbow room, between himself and that with which others assume he should be identified" (1961:319). Goffman scrutinized the total institution from the point of view of the group as well as from the point of view of the individual. Unlike most social theorists before him, he questioned the harmonious, functionalist fit between the two social entities. He also observed discrepancies between official expectations and the actual responses by participants: "We find that participants decline in some way to accept the official view of what they should be putting into and getting out of the organization and, behind this, of what sort of self and world they are to accept for themselves. Where enthusiasm is expected, there will be apathy; where loyalty, there will be disaffection; where attendance, absenteeism; where robustness, some kind of illness; where deeds are to be done, varieties of inactivity. We find a multitude of homely little histories, each in its way a movement of liberty. Whenever worlds are laid on, underlives develop" (1961:304–5).

Noting that every institution has "encompassing" tendencies, he isolated five types of "total" institutions.[4] While Goffman understood that variety exists among total institutions, and though he included old-age homes in his scheme, he did not provide illustrations of them.

Structural Features and Resident Response

The characteristics of total institutions are divided into structural features of the institution and the responses of inmates (Table 3). Whereas people normally sleep, eat, work, and socialize in different places, these behaviors are in one place in the total institution. This structural characteristic fits the case of Franklin. Activities are scheduled according to plans administered within the institution. Residents are generally treated alike though a competing philosophy of care insists that residents are unique individuals. Nonperson treatment, examined below, is a standard of resident care at Franklin. The moral order of the total institution, as Goffman saw it, includes a usually latent and pervasive component. The moral order sustains itself, and an inmate of a total institution becomes molded into and equated with it as he passes through the admission process. In Goffman's example,

[97]

Table 3. Characteristics of total institutions

Characteristics	Present at Franklin
Structural aspects	
All activities in one place	Yes
People treated in group	Yes
Activities brought together	Yes
Split between inmates and staff	Yes
Make-work (activities)	Yes
Information control	Yes
Nonperson treatment	Yes
Stripping and mortification	Partially
Clean break with past	Partially
Privilege and punishment system	No
Role releases	Yes
Returned to society	No
Moral order	Yes
Inmate response	
Collective teasing	Partially
Feeling of personal failure	Partially
Stigmatization	Partially
Knowing the ropes	Partially
Inmate fraternalization	Partially

admission to a mental hospital defines the individual as a mental patient who requires mental service. In the case of this nursing home, admission means that the old person is unable to care for himself given whatever outside resources he does (and does not) have. The institutionalized old person is equated with a dependent child. Goffman writes: "While many individuals can be relied upon to act as responsible, self-willing agents in regard to their bodies, it is apparent that the very young, the very old, and the mentally ill may have to be brought to medical attention 'for their own good' by someone else, thus radically changing the usual relation between client, possession, and server" (1961:344). Though residents and staff make some attempt to blur the distinction between them, as in the employee-versus-friend dichotomy, the division in status between them is of lasting importance. Official information is always closely regulated, especially regarding firing and deaths. Residents devise their own strategies for gaining information, given the restrictions on official information flow. Though occupational therapy is often considered by the most intact residents to be superfluous and not of real value, all residents seem to appreciate how these activities kill time.

The partial nature of stripping behaviors and those that facilitate making a clean break with the past in this nursing home result from specific institutional factors and resident responses to institutionalization. Individuals have to "break up" their homes and relinquish many past roles and belongings when they enter the nursing home. Some retain ties with the outside, and some have few or no ties to maintain. Though a person must relinquish his home and most of his belongings, including his driver's license, he need not wear institutional clothing, have his hair cut, or undergo other leveling procedures typical in total institutions, except that he must wear the resented identification wristbands. Gubrium has commented: "To many residents, wearing these bands is demeaning. After all, they consider themselves to be *residents* in the Manor, not patients, as in a hospital. They are very alert to the distinction. Most residents have grumbled about the wrist band requirement at one time or another" (1975:102).

Goffman described at length various adaptations that inmates make to the institution. Franklin residents share some of these inmate-response characteristics (Table 3). The most intact residents sometimes criticize staff members in a teasing manner. They note jealousies and jockeyings for power among staff and are amused. Some residents are ashamed to be in the nursing home and are loath to use the name of the nursing home as an address. Others do not feel this way at all and accept the nursing home residence with aplomb and resignation. Residents devise strategies, as accommodations to the nursing home, to manipulate staff, obtain information, have favors fulfilled, and subvert inconvenient rules. Finally, regarding fraternalization, residents get along with each other in some ways, but in many ways maintain isolated patterns of being "good patients" and remain docile and quiet.

Two important features of institutional behaviors—privilege and punishment and returning to the outside—are not found at Franklin. There is little expectation that a resident, once admitted to this nursing home, will be reinstated in the community. It is for this reason that a privilege and punishment system makes no sense. Not only are privilege and punishment systems set up for institutional control of inmates, they are also the mechanisms by which inmates secure their release from the total institution. Entrance to this nursing home, however, indicates that the deteriorating downhill course of an aged

[99]

individual will continue to worsen until death. Though there is debate within the administration of the nursing home about admitting people for more rehabilitative and short-term stays, most residents remain in the nursing home until death.

People-Work

People-work is a vital feature of total institutions and is characteristic of the work at Franklin. Goffman describes people-work thus:

> [There is often a contradiction] between what the institution does and what its officials must say it does, [and this contradiction] forms the basic context of the staff's daily activity. Within this context, perhaps the first thing to say about the staff is that their work, and hence their world, have uniquely to do with people. This *people-work* is not quite like personnel work or the work of those involved in service relationships; the staff, after all, have objects and products to work upon, not services, but these objects and products are people. As material upon which to work, people can take on somewhat the same characteristics as inanimate objects. Surgeons prefer to operate on slender patients rather than fat ones, because with fat ones instruments get slippery, and there are the extra layers to cut through. (1961:74, Goffman's italics)

This aspect of resident care is manifest in all areas of the nursing home, but is primarily evident in the work that nursing assistants and orderlies do. Bodies have specific problems of management. Heavy bodies require more than one nursing assistant or orderly to lift; incontinent bodies require frequent toileting; "superblends" require being fed blended food; and so on. Though the resident may want most of all to talk with the nursing assistant for companionship and the alleviation of loneliness, the nursing assistant's perception of her job is to make sure that her resident is bathed, toileted, and fed on time so that she will be able to perform similar duties on her other residents. If the nursing assistant neglects to clean the resident's fingernails, she will be blamed. Therefore, a nursing assistant may be impatient with her resident at mealtime if the resident wants to talk or is eating with her fingers after her nails were cleaned. Ensuring that certain standards of the organization are kept is the main priority. The resident's chest of drawers must be cleaned regularly; the resident's person must be maintained so that should an administrator happen by, or should the state decide to have an inspection that day, such matters will have been handled properly.

People-work considerations thus relate directly to the nonperson treatment afforded the aged in institutions. People-work also determines the principle that "persons are almost always considered to be ends in themselves" (Goffman 1961:76). As such, they are objects to be preserved. Residents' intentions to hasten their deaths must be thwarted. Some nurses expressed to me their preference for residents for whom they could perform "real nursing." They liked the skilled-nursing floors better than the intermediate-care floors because there are more procedures to perform. When specific nursing tasks are not called for, many nurses say their skills are not being utilized, and they are bored. Chart work and staffing take priority over talking to the residents when specific nursing tasks are not pressing. Like Gubrium's descriptions of "bed and body work" in Murray Manor, the work that nursing assistants and orderlies do on the bodies of Franklin residents goes on separately from considerations of the persons who inhabit those bodies. Because the persons are effectively separated from their bodies, these procedures are promulgated as ends in themselves. People-work routines therefore contribute to the repetitive, here and now, timelessness that cycles through every day of the nursing home.

Limitations of Goffman's Model

Most nursing homes are not rigid in the ways that Goffman described. In the same way that individuals in Goffman's model scramble to subvert the rules and regulations of encompassing institutions, so too perhaps do individual organizations depart from the ideal total institution.

Goffman's model makes no allowance for total institutions with competing ideologies of care. Hierarchies that operate within the bureaucracy, each with its own territorialities, worldviews, and modi operandi, create undulating tensions that prevent unity—prevent the totality of total institutions. Administrators contend with the need for budget cuts at the same time that they want to show their contributors in the community how up-to-date and complete their services to the elderly are. The home-hospital dichotomy pits staff member against staff member, and frequent life versus quality-of-life decisions challenge staff members to cooperate in the residents' interests. The rehabilitation philosophy struggles against that of maintenance and surfaces in treatment routines and the pursuit of daily activities.

Goffman likewise did not consider the heterogeneous population served by the total institution—the clientele or the inmates. Demonstrating how significant it is that these institutions operate as if all inmates were the same, he did not explore the actual heterogeneity of inmate populations within one institution. At Franklin there are three main groups of residents with separate, sometimes competing, needs. These categories are not necessarily the same as the level-of-care designations that the state makes for each resident.

One group is composed of extremely ill or debilitated individuals. They are unable to fulfill any of their physical needs, but they may be capable of understanding and communicating. The second group, the largest group in the nursing home, is composed of those residents who are considered demented and may or may not be physically capable of certain activities. A resident in this group might be anxious, wander through the premises, cry out at night, and not remember where he is, yet at the same time, he may be able to dress himself, feed himself, and toilet himself. He may need little nursing care beyond some supervision and guidance. Another confused resident may have trouble dressing herself, have periods of clarity in which she understands that her mind is failing, may be depressed and isolated, but may need varying amounts of physical help and emotional support. Thus, even the members of this group cannot be treated alike. The third group consists of those residents who are considered the most capable, both physically and mentally, but they are heterogeneous in their needs for support, medication, and so forth. By and large, the individuals in this group remain separate from the other two groups. This separation derives both from their own wishes and from institutional provisions that aid separation.

These groups, fairly distinct and with quite separate needs, are contained in the same institution. Nursing-home personnel at times try to treat people individually, but they also treat them as if their needs were similar. Goffman noted how total institutions attempt to homogenize their inmates, but he did not deal with how the total institution is diluted by the heterogeneity that always exists. Because there are competing staff goals, as well as three different resident groups in the nursing home, myriad responses are created. In short, the monolithic institution is not so monolithic.

Other total institutions share characteristics similar to those of the Franklin Nursing Home; therefore the critique of Goffman's model is pertinent to them as well. Mental hospitals and jails have staff members who espouse conflicting ideologies regarding how to treat inmates. Further, other total institutions have heterogeneous populations; jails and mental hospitals incarcerate people of varying degrees of danger to themselves and others, and staff members must distinguish among the inmates in order to provide care, maintain order, and assure safety.

Goffman described an adversarial relationship between staff and inmates, which he says periodically breaks down in "role releases" when the inmate-staff split is either blurred, erased, or reversed. He neglected to explain why this adversarial relationship exists, especially in nursing homes where the staff is supposed to serve the residents. He described the inmate-staff split, and left it at that. When people are incarcerated against their wills, it is intuitively understandable that antagonism exists. Why a similar antipathy might develop in nursing homes is not so apparent.

Some of the answer might be found in a closer examination of the competing themes in the nursing home both from the points of view of staff members and of residents. Goffman implies, though does not develop, the idea that the experience of being in a total institution is similar to that of a rite of passage. He notes that inmates have been degraded in status, that they have been stripped of their past roles, and that they are like social infants who have to be socialized to their new role. He also alludes to the fact that inmates' ability to contribute is derailed in the total institution.

Many of the traits of total institutions, therefore, translate into reciprocity and/or into rites-of-passage terms. However, these factors remain descriptive rather than analytical, and static rather than processual, and therefore fail to illuminate certain contradictory and dynamic elements. For example, what Goffman describes as stripping, mortification, and separation correspond easily to separation in rites-of-passage theory. Various words that Goffman uses to describe the adaptation of inmates to their institutionalized state translate into what van Gennep or Turner would call the liminal or transitional state. Notions such as make-do's, underlife, secondary adjustment, moral order, people-work, people as ends in themselves, resident fraternalization, and role releases all describe aspects of liminality in the rite of passage. Finally, privilege and punishment and returning to the outside correspond to reincorporation in rites of passage. However, Goffman's terminology and description falls short in the domain of liminality. The notion of liminality encompasses contradictions and ambiguities that Goffman's terms cannot handle. Goffman's terminology is too cut-and-dried; the competing strains and tensions among personnel of the total institution are not elaborated with their processual complexities. There is little sense of movement, of evolution. Rather, the total institution is described as a certain structural concept with determining characteristics; inmates are portrayed as having embattled selves, which are assaulted by the domination of the total institution; and inmates and staff are shown to devise strategies to combat each other and function together. The total institution is simplified.

The Franklin Nursing Home is a total institution, but quite unlike those Goffman described. It is not merely a bureaucracy with competing ideological hierarchies. It is a home where comforts, companionship, continuity, and individuality are inhibited. It is a hospital, but no one is cured of the ailment that brought him to it, frail old age. Because there is no consensus about goals for the residents, staff members work against one another. Because the residents are heterogeneous, they are not exactly like initiates who share the same experience. Because they are treated like incapable children, their individualities and their pasts are denied them, they are unable to contribute, and they must be grateful for the care they receive. This status sometimes incites resentment among staff. It clearly exacerbates the powerlessness of residents, which was already well initiated before admission. Residents are in a rite of passage from adulthood to death which has been interrupted midstream. In the following chapters, I develop these ideas of the nursing home as a place where reciprocity is structurally prohibited for the inmates and where each individual embarks on a singular rite of passage that is stripped of its ritual solidarity and symbolic meanings.

Notebook:
5:00 A.M.–10:00 A.M.

When I get to the home this morning, I introduce myself to the security guard on duty at the front desk. He offers to unlock the social service office so that I can leave my pocketbook in there. The nursing home is darkened.

It's a freezing morning. In the front lobby I see Mr. Roitman reading the newspaper. He tells me he's waiting for the morning orthodox services, which will start around 6:00 A.M. or so. Today he'll be going out to buy new pants. His wife is not doing well: "She is in God's hands now," he says. I usually see them together, walking hand in hand down the corridors. She always appears anxious; her face tilts up in bewilderment and consternation. He greets people in the halls; she tugs at his arm, and he sometimes looks aggrieved and irritated. She lives in the main building because she requires more care, but she searches him out everyday, and he says he wishes she would leave him alone more often. "She's not right, you know, in her head. She used to be mean and now she's usually nice, but sometimes she's mean and hits the nurses or the aides. Then she gets terribly upset and apologetic. The nurses can't hit back." "That's good," I comment, and I'm surprised that he looks up, rather startled, as if he's puzzled that it's unfair that they don't have the right to retaliate.

I excuse myself to wander around the building before the morning services begin. I go up to the second floor of the new building. It's dark except for the night lights lining the halls. I introduce myself to the charge nurse at the nurses' station. She says it has been a quiet night. During the night one can detect changes, tell if someone's sick. For example, a person who usually sleeps well was screaming one night, and it developed that she had pneumonia. Some nights are noisy because people cry out or yell. Many of the residents become used to it; in fact, one resident with Alzheimer's was troubled after her noisy roommate moved out. She couldn't sleep because she'd become accustomed to the noise.

I go to the second floor wing. It is also dark. As I go down the hall someone comes out of a resident's room and asks if I need help. I introduce myself. She is dressed in white and I can't make out more than that. She approaches me. She is a short, round woman with gray hair that sticks up around her head. At first, I can't understand what she is saying or whether she's a resident or a staff person.

Her name is Mabel Johnson and she has worked nights on this floor for many years. She was just now taking Minnie to the bathroom and just before that she had been in Ettie Wood's room because Ettie is depressed after having come back from the hospital following heart surgery. "They have a fit when I'm not here," she tells me in a very quiet voice, full of understatement. She tells me that she does little kind things "secretlike," without attracting official notice. As we talk, I feel myself adoring this woman. She describes how the residents are lonely and how she feels she should help them. Her voice is smooth and low, measured, soothing. When someone cannot sleep at night, she says, "Well, maybe you took too long a nap during the afternoon, so why don't you get up and have some warm milk and watch TV with me; that'll be okay." She comforts them this way. She holds and soothes them. She took care of her mother, who lived a very long time, and she says that to live to the ages of these people is a blessing. It's as if they are holy to have been blessed with such long lives, and her work to make them comfortable is a way of honoring them. When I leave her, she hugs and kisses me, and I do the same to her. I feel like I've met a beautiful apparition in the dark. She seems to embody caring and warmth in the night.

I go quickly to the third floor of the new building, and introduce myself to the charge nurse there. She tells me that the night has been fine, but quite busy. "We have a lot of wetters on this floor, a lot of wetters." Therefore the nursing assistants and orderlies are busy changing the residents every two hours. Catheters are not allowed on this floor at night.

Some of the residents are up. One of the men who come to the home to participate in services is helping a man get ready to go downstairs to the chapel. I'm told that some of the other men have already gone.

I go downstairs for the services. About a dozen people are in the shul, *having coffee. I meet Mr. Werner, who leads the services. Another man hands me coffee and presses a donut on me. The services used to begin at 5:30, but they've been pushed ahead to a time more convenient for the residents. It is difficult to assemble the necessary minyan [a quorum of ten men over age 13] for these services so Mr. Werner offers coffee and doughnuts and recruits men from the community to join them. I'm told the services will begin in fifteen minutes. I decide I have time to check on the fourth floor.*

Up there I'm told that it was a noisy night. Maybe it's a full moon, the nurse suggests. She says that everyone was up; there was much dreaming and screaming, and those who were noisy woke those who had been sleeping. They just had their flu shots yesterday; maybe that was it. I go back down to the shul.

Some of the men are wrapping tfilin *on their arms. A man with a paralyzed arm asks one of the men from the community to help him with his. The resident communicates by gestures and grunting; he cannot speak. The man from the community gruffly challenges me to identify these ritual objects. He seems surprised that I correctly identify the various parts of dress. He tells me that there are all kinds of people in here. "This man used to be a lawyer. This man a tailor, this man a furniture salesman." As he is talking, he shows me his bare forearm with the number tatooed on it. I tell him that I'd noticed it. I ask him where, and he shushes me and walks away. A few minutes later he comes back, and he says he was in Auschwitz and Buchenwald, "some of those nice hotels," as he puts it. He came here in 1949. He prays at the nursing home because it's early and it's close by.*

A woman comes into the service. I recognize her as Sadie Berman. She sits across the aisle from Mr. Roitman. The man from the community points her out to me and says that she came in here and lost her mind a little. That has been my impression as well.

While the service is going on, the man from the community is walking to and fro, and when it comes to the memorial parts, he raises his voice very loud. They usually have about twelve people at the service. The afternoon service at 4:30 attracts more. Mr. Roitman was begged to come to the morning services. He used to read his paper in the hall and didn't want to come in. They cajoled him with the coffee and their need to have the minyan.

Mrs. Berman whispers loudly to Mr. Roitman about me: "Who is she?" He tells her my name. He tells her I have a husband. "Where is he?" she fires back. I smile to myself.

The man from the community now goes up the aisle with a box for collections. He extends the box ceremoniously to me, but I don't have my pocketbook with me. He admonishes me, "Next time!" After the service is over, I explain that I'd left my pocketbook in the locked-up office. Quizzing me about my temple membership and our religious observances, he challenges me to tell him how we educate our children to know about tradition, history, and sacrifice. He seems somewhat satisfied by my complicated explanation.

Mr. Werner says that the nursing home doesn't care about the services and that if he wasn't there, there wouldn't be any morning services at all. "And the old people don't care either," he adds. I ask why. He thinks they've given up; also, most people are not orthodox anymore. He shrugs his shoulders with resignation. Everyone is leaving now. It is about 7:15.

I go up to the second floor, which is now lit. One of the nurses has accidentally locked her keys in the medication closet. The director of nurses has been called as well as the security guard. The security man pretends he doesn't have the keys and jokes with everyone about her locking the door. I ask him how the night was. He answers that it was a quiet night, but that it's often very busy. Sometimes they have breaking and entering attempts.

The orderly, Hal, comes in. Sayzie asks why he's late, and he goes through a long, wearied story about how he sold his car and how he just missed the bus, and the bus driver actually looked at him as he drove by. Today's charge nurse, Ellie, comes into the nurses' station, and just as Hal is sitting down, she says, "Don't sit down, Hal; it's 7:30." He gives her a sullen look and says something like "Cut it out— you're not gonna bug me again today, are you?" But she insists, saying, "Get going; I mean it Hal," and looks worn and resigned. She and I exchange looks. It's tense. She once described how she has to push everyone to do anything. Ellie had told me that she didn't think she could keep working here very long.

Jeanine jokes that if I'm writing about her, she's going to hit me. I mention the day I followed Aymara around, and the memory makes everyone moan. Now Jeanine says that she got approval from downstairs that Halloween decorations are going to be okay this year! Hal says, "Jeez, why not! Good reality orientation, right?" sarcastically. Sayzie says that the objections had something to do with the Catholic origins of the holiday. That explanation produces a give-me-a-break groan from someone. I suddenly wonder what it would be like to have these people take care of me.

The buzzer sounds. They look to the board to identify the person. "It's Edie," says Sayzie. "Probably wants to get off the toilet. Probably wants to know if she's gone."

Spotting Charlie Kassin, I ask him if he's making his daily rounds and if I can join him. He seems pleased. The food trucks are already coming up, though the residents won't be eating for a while. The food trucks stay plugged in to keep warm. Mr. Kassin and I walk from the new building to the wing. He looks chipper and says he's fine—why not, his usual. We chat with a few nurses, then Mr. Kassin goes on his way. I go to the third floor to look for Sarah Zeldin. I tell her about the nursing assistant I met here hours ago in the dark. "Oh," says Mrs. Zeldin, meaningfully, "Mabel Johnson." Mrs. Zeldin knows her well. She'd had fourteen children. That doesn't surprise me. Mrs. Zeldin and I have a nice long visit.

Notebook:
Resident-Care Conference

Three residents will be presented today. Charlie Rosenbaum, 82, is obese and difficult to manage. He never married. When he was admitted six years ago, he weighed 300 pounds. Now, he weighs about 230. He may have some dementia, though maybe he's just depressed. Dr. Corning comments that sometimes the person knows the answers to the mental status test but doesn't care about the answers, and sometimes the depression is actually causing the person not to know.

Present today are several nurses, a dietician, the activities director, a few social workers, and me. The dietician says that Mr. Rosenbaum steals food from other people's trays. To remedy this problem, he is now eating by himself. Dr. Corning asks, "What do you mean, 'steal'?" She explains that he takes the food from those who are confused; at other times he throws his tray at people. He loves his cigars, attends no activities, and watches TV. He fights with Jacob Strauss at least once a day, but no one present at the meeting seems to think that there is anything wrong with that since Mr. Strauss is hard to get along with.

Mr. Rosenbaum is shown in with his nursing assistant, and the interview is very short. Dr. Corning asks him about being sad. Mr. Rosenbaum says that he doesn't think anything can be done about it. The nursing assistant has nothing to add. After some long silences, Dr. Corning tells him he can go.

Lisa, the social worker, now presents Mrs. Kaplan. She was abused as a child and was raised by her grandparents after she was 9. Her father was alcoholic and beat her, and the mother was unsympathetic. Of Mrs. Kaplan's three children, one daughter visits every day. Mrs.

Kaplan has been chronically depressed since her husband died in 1949. When Lisa asked her what year it was for the mental status exam, she answered 1949. She is 85 years old, American born.

The daughter comes in with questions ready. She knows that her mother is difficult, but couldn't she get her hair done sometimes? It would make her feel better. Louise, the nurse, says that it's hard to get an appointment and to transport her. As the daughter insists, Dr. Corning pronounces it done. Next: couldn't her mother go to more parties in the home? She knows her mother usually doesn't want to go and cries, but the daughter thinks it would be beneficial. Discussion reveals that she does go to parties. Next: mother's teeth were stolen, and couldn't she get some new ones? The daughter knows that things "walk" here and there, but her mother would like some new teeth. Also, her mother isn't really incontinent, and the daughter is upset when she sees her mother in a diaper. Can't they ask her a little more often if she has to use the toilet, because if they ask her, she will go. Louise explains that diapers are used more frequently on the 3:00 P.M. to 11:00 P.M. shift because there are fewer staff people on duty then, but the daughter says that the diaper is on at times during the day shift as well.

She says that she thinks her mother should be treated more like a person, and it makes her mad to hear staff members sometimes say things like "so and so is really crazy; he or she should be put away." Her mother has the fear that she will be sent away. The daughter believes that a staff member must have suggested the possibility to her mother. "I know there are a lot of sick people here, and I know my mother isn't easy, but this is a place for sick people, isn't it?" finishes the daughter with exasperation.

Lisa responds that she understands that the daughter can calm her mother's frequent crying spells. The daughter says that she used to be able to calm her, but no longer. Now her mother complains and cries more when she comes. She doesn't take her out anymore because the mother immediately wants to come back or screams in the car. The daughter seems on the verge of tears.

Mrs. Kaplan is shown in. She is barely understandable because she has no teeth. She is asked if she would like teeth. Yes. Is everything else okay? No, not the roommate. The daughter remembers something else: her mother's eyes are a problem. Mrs. Kaplan is asked about this and says she can't see out of either eye. She is assured that there will be a check-up in the new eye clinic very soon. As Mrs. Kaplan is shown

[111]

out, the daughter promises her mother that she'll be up to her room soon. Everyone agrees that Mrs. Kaplan was lucid during the meeting. The daughter is reassured that the staff will make some changes. Dr. Corning thanks her for the good questions and input.

As the daughter leaves, Louise immediately blurts, "It's going to be impossible to bring that lady down to get her hair done; I don't know how we're ever going to do it." Bernice says, "She was lucid? I could barely understand her." A few staff members share anecdotes about how difficult she is to manage and how she hollers. A social worker says that a long time ago she was a dental assistant and she knows about the process of making impressions for false teeth. It's involved, takes time, causes discomfort, and after the teeth are made and in, they often hurt. She is convinced that this woman would never wear her new teeth.

Dr. Corning looks surprised and exasperated. "Wait a minute, wait a minute, one person talk at a time. Why wasn't any of this brought up while she was here?" He goes on to express his belief that the family members are necessary in the interdisciplinary concept of this meeting and that when the daughter had suggestions, it was dishonest and counterproductive not to provide the information that is now emerging about why or why not the suggestions were appropriate. So now the staff is in the ridiculous position of having agreed to things that are either difficult or impossible to carry out, and it will seem that the staff doesn't get things done, or lies, both of which the daughter believes already. Each staff member is defensive about why she didn't offer the information she had. The former dental assistant says that teeth is nursing, not a part of her expertise. Dr. Corning says no, she had that experience, and it was her obligation to provide her informed opinion. Dr. Corning says the daughter needed to be confronted in a nice way in this setting. A nurse says that they'll arrange the dental consult and then they'll be off the hook because he'll probably recommend what they're saying anyhow. And they will get the hair done once anyhow. But it will be difficult, not only because of personnel needed to transport her down and back up again but because the hairdresser usually insists that the nursing assistant stay with the resident to transfer her to the proper chair. All of this takes time and people. Everyone suddenly seems weary.

Next, Harriet now presents Mrs. Williams. Her dementia began ten years ago when she was only 60 years old. An Ivy League college graduate, she held top administrative jobs in the region. She retired eight years ago because of the dementia and was admitted here three years later. Her four children live elsewhere and do not visit. Her husband divorced her and has remarried, but remains devoted to her, visiting her often. She knows no one, is on total nursing care, and sometimes laughs to herself. Her medical problems are listed as: Alzheimer's disease, seizure disorder, cerebral arterial insufficiency.

There's an undertone of discussion about the husband's having remarried. Was this a proper thing for him to do? Bernice mutters: the children were against it. She adds "till death do us part," for emphasis. Harriet argues that it is healthier to do what he did than to deny the reality and ruin his own life as well. There is a lot of feeling about this issue. Gloria, the activities director, asks me why I'm quiet and wants to know what I think. I say that I think the husband behaved properly, but that I can't imagine what it must be like. Dr. Corning agrees that the husband did the right thing, but his wife better not ever do that to him! This produces some welcome laughter.

Mrs. Williams is now wheeled into the staff room. She's a handsome woman with grayish white hair. Her head angles up stiffly and awkwardly. She seems unseeing and is unresponsive to what Dr. Corning says to her. He strokes her hair from her forehead back in a soothing and firm motion. She mumbles something unintelligible and laughs quietly. Dr. Corning asks her nursing assistant if Mrs. Williams understands her at any time, but the nursing assistant responds that she doesn't think so. Dr. Corning lets them leave. There is quiet talk. Mrs. Williams has affected everyone. The woman looks intelligent still; her facial features are refined and chiseled precisely. She looks young. Top administrator. Everyone seems moved.

The meeting is over. I go out with one of the social workers, who says, "How could there even be an issue about whether the husband's behavior was 'right' or not!" She tells me that there is a man administering to his wife in the home at the present. He's constantly there, hovering, doing. She thinks he will fall apart when the woman dies. His behavior makes no sense to her. Life should go on, she mutters adamantly.

[6]

Bridges to the Community

Not really a part of, and not totally separated from the Harrison community, Franklin is at a certain symbolic distance from the city. A person entering the nursing home leaves the community in significant ways. But bridging the separation between the institution and Harrison are certain ameliorating features, which are tenuous, unclear, shifting, and not often synchronized with each other. Whereas some nursing homes contain an in-house medical staff, Harrison physicians—with outside practices—constitute an ambiguously defined bridge to the community. The local hospital, the Jewish community and its fund-raising sector, the board of trustees, and the volunteers who donate time to the nursing home likewise both connect the nursing home to the community and maintain a separateness between them.

The Medical Community

Though Franklin is affiliated with a local medical school and a gerontology center, the administration of the nursing home has reservations about the association and prefers to be more autonomous and separate. For example, though there is willingness to conduct research and to open the nursing home to students, some of the research is considered esoteric and possibly jeopardizing to the status quo.[1] Medical students and medical residents circulate through the building increasingly, but their ideas and suggestions are sometimes interpreted as academic rather than useful.

[114]

Physicians are at the summit of the medical hierarchy in the nursing home, but they are an infrequent presence. Mitchell and Hewes (1986) have attempted to document physicians' reasons for not visiting nursing-home patients. Reasons include reimbursement difficulties, distaste for nursing homes, inefficient use of time, and other factors. Seventy-two percent of private-practice physicians do not make nursing-home visits (Mitchell 1982). Their absence creates logistical difficulties and resentment within the nursing home. The part-time medical director encapsulates the bridging role of the physicians whose patients are in Franklin. He oversees medical matters within the nursing home. He visits his own patients; he directs and attends meetings that relate to resident care, circumstances of death, prospective admissions, policy questions, organizational management, relations with the union, and long-range planning. In acting as a liaison between the nursing home and the private physicians whose patients are residents, he must tactfully remind reluctant physicians to make their regular visits. He feels he softens his official role as medical director, for he is a practicing physician in the community like his colleagues. Other nursing homes have solved this dual-role problem by having a medical staff on salary. This situation enables the formulation of explicit rules and duties of the employee physicians. It also ensures that physicians are on the premises; it facilitates having a pharmacy within the institution; it eliminates the tension that exists for nurses who must phone physicians about residents' problems. Furthermore, a full-time medical director need not be concerned about referrals from the community.[2]

When residents are admitted to Franklin, they used to retain their former physicians (see note 2). Medicare and Medicaid regulations stipulate how often residents must be seen by their physicians, depending on their level of care.[3] Meshing the shadowy actual presence of the physician with the legal prominence that the physician holds constituted one of the major logistical struggles that occured daily within the institution during fieldwork. The following is an example of a common problem that results from the insufficient presence of physicians on the nursing-home premises:

A resident has begun getting out of a chair that he used to sit in quietly for long periods of time. Upon rising, he often becomes dizzy and then falls. The orderly who is assigned to this resident complains to the charge nurse on his shift that the resident's behavior has changed. The orderly feels that the resident is in danger. Furthermore, the orderly does not want to injure himself lifting the resident often. The nurse phones the physician but is unable to reach him. She telephones again later, but again is unsuccessful. He does not return her call. Meanwhile, the resident's daughter has come to visit, and is upset that her father has fallen a few times. She wants something to be done. The orderly who is on duty during another shift is not aware of the change in the resident. The orderly has had the last two days off and does not know what has happened in the meantime. He tells the resident's daughter that her father is fine. The following day the physician telephones a different nurse and orders a restraining chair for the resident (called a geriatric or "gerry" chair). Some of the personnel on duty follow the doctor's orders, and some of them do not.

There is often a lag between a change in a resident's behavior and the medical response. The resident may resent the geriatric chair and may fight, kick, and bite his orderly. Possibly, careful monitoring of the resident could substitute for the need for the geriatric chair, but an increase in staffing would be required. Therefore, use of the geriatric chair is often one of convenience and expediency. The physician may not want to issue orders that he knows the nursing staff are reluctant to institute. The combination of the absent physician and the personnel on the nursing shifts who insufficiently communicate with each other impedes consistent care.

Residents opinions of physicians are varied. Though residents sometimes complain that they see their doctors too infrequently, most of them have a long-term relationship with their physicians, and they view the doctors with fondness and some reverence. Family members, acting as consumer advocates, often press physicians for information and alternate modes of care. Another fairly prevalent attitude among residents is the feeling that doctors can do little to improve their situations. Physicians and residents both seem to know that chronic and accumulating ailments will not yield easily to medical intervention, and if they do, new problems will undoubtably arise. Nursing-home residents might not be bitter that their doctors come infrequently if their visits were more purely social rather than cursorily palliative. Physicians, however, may avoid visiting their nursing-home patients because they know, and dislike knowing, that there is little they can do.

The relationship between the neighboring hospital (where Franklin residents are almost invariably hospitalized) and the nursing home is the result of certain historical factors and is also marked by separation and closeness. Located near each other, the hospital and the nursing home have evolved along parallel lines through the years, both institutions maintaining contact and autonomy at the same time. Since the creation of the university's medical school, the quality of the hospital has improved dramatically. In response to the fact that half of the hospital's patient population is over the age of 65, the hospital has a nurse-practitioner on its staff. The physicians at the hospital are the same ones whose patients are at the nursing home. The nursing and social-worker staffs of the two institutions are separate, however. Nurses at the hospital have more power and input into medical decisions than do the nurses at the nursing home. Notwithstanding the fact that the two nursing staffs have great overlap in their patient population, there is little communication between them and a frequent amount of misunderstanding. For example:

The nurses at Franklin are proud that most of their residents are up and around and that the bane of nursing homes, bedsores (decubitus ulcers), is a rare occurrence here. They are dismayed that the nurses at the hospital assume that poor nursing practices go on at the nursing home. When a patient returns from the hospital with a bedsore, both the hospital and nursing home personnel claim the bedsore was acquired at the other's facility. The nurses at the hospital are not always able to keep the aged patients active. The residents from the nursing home arrive at the hospital during an acute, usually life-threatening episode. The hospital nurses do not have the opportunity to witness these same individuals in their previous, more healthy state, and they assume a lower mode of functioning for these patients. Therefore, according to Franklin nurses, the hospital nurses expect less of these patients and return them to the nursing home at a reduced level of health.

The hospital nurses consider the nursing done at the nursing home to be inferior, custodial care. This belief is different from the reality. The nursing done at Franklin is arduous and specialized. Geriatric nursing requires extensive knowledge and experience. Syndromes manifest themselves differently in aged patients and middle-aged ones; psychosocial issues are different; many procedures, such as finding veins in aged patients to do bloodwork, require an exactness not necessary for younger patients.

Misunderstanding between the personnel of the hospital and the nursing home accompanies the immense traffic that goes on between the two institutions. While geriatric education of medical students is taking place and the local gerontology center is having an impact, permeation of geriatric knowledge throughout the medical and nursing establishments in the region has only just begun.

Leadership and Funding

The board of trustees oversees the organization of the nursing home. It conducts the search for the executive officers of the nursing home; it hires the new administrator; it determines the overall operation of the nursing home. Its decisions determine admission policies and plans for the future.

The Jewish Federation in Harrison has made up the deficit of the nursing home for the last several years. Several Jewish organizations in the area compete for funds from the largest Jewish funding body. This competition impedes cooperation between the organizations. Jewish leadership in the community is divided over the future direction of the nursing home. Issues have had to do with the nursing home's relationship to the medical school, the gerontology center, and the university, as well as with its ties to the hospital. Should apartment housing for graduated long-term care be constructed? Where should it be? Who should constitute the population of the nursing home? Should the nursing home care only for the very sick and very poor aged, or should an attempt be made to offer various kinds of care and services to a more heterogeneous resident population? At one time, the community was divided over plans to move the nursing home. Population projections indicated that the Jewish population was moving to the suburbs, closer to highways and malls. Some leaders argued that a rural setting was preferable for the aged population. Another plan was to construct an apartment complex for the elderly within the city near the existing Jewish organizations and synagogues. But there was no unity. The result was that the sheltered apartment complex was built in the suburbs, and the nursing home remained where it was, in proximity to the hospital and the Jewish organizations. In all, there is little consensus on the decisions facing the future of the nursing home.

Volunteers

Volunteer assistance at the nursing home is also marked by ambiguity and ambivalence. For example, though the Women's Federation is active in raising funds for the institution, few of its members are involved personally with the residents. Similarly, Franklin was to be a religious haven for aged Jews, but there is little interaction between the religious community outside the nursing home and the residents.[4]

There has been difficulty in finding a rabbi to come to the nursing home. There is no rabbi at the home's orthodox, early morning daily services. At the end of my fieldwork, the nursing home sent a letter to all of the area congregations asking each to be responsible for a month at the nursing home—for example, to be present in some capacity for Friday evening services. Most of the congregations have agreed to this plan, and there has been more community participation as a result.[5]

Individual volunteers are usually students, homemakers, or the retired. They do "friendly visiting" with the residents, help transport residents to activities, mend clothes, or do other tasks. Some Jewish educational organizations are involved in the nursing home. The Hillel chapter of the local universities encourages students to visit the residents. Sometimes the local Hebrew schools present programs for the residents, and a nearby nursery school has made occasional visits. Nonetheless, a sentiment among the Jewish staff at the nursing home is that the Jewish community of Harrison avoids personal involvement in the home, preferring to limit its activity to the financial.[6] Frequently, too, volunteers who want to help are discouraged to do so by the employees, who at other times complain of staffing shortages.

The nurse was telling me that better coordination would help. If she could have a regular volunteer to do some of the paperwork that plagues her, she would find the service useful. But there isn't enough continuity among the volunteers. Or if she could count on a few people to show up at certain times to transport residents to their activities, that would be good, too. Sometimes a volunteer will suddenly show up; but without advance notice, the nurse is simply too busy to spend time with the volunteer thinking of things that the volunteer could do.

[119]

Difficulty in coordinating volunteers and staff thus prevent good utilization of some of the community resources that are available. Furthermore, the union bristles at volunteers who are too helpful.

A middle-aged volunteer was found to be an enthusiastic and energetic worker who had a history of mental problems and a low tolerance for stressful situations. He wanted to help out within the nursing home because he needed a way to structure his time. The director of volunteers assigned him to janitorial work because he loved to clean things, and he was found to be meticulous and hard working. After he had worked for a few weeks, the regular housekeeping staff complained to the administration that if this volunteer was not removed, they would complain to the union. The housekeeping staff felt that this volunteer worked so hard and so well that his example would undermine hard-won guidelines determining their job descriptions. They would be expected to work as well. The result was that the volunteer was moved to the kitchen, but he eventually left because kitchen work was too stressful for him.

Connections between Franklin and the Harrison community are numerous, but they are difficult, riddled by ambivalence, and marked by territoriality and competition. These factors isolate the nursing home so that when elderly individuals are admitted, they leave community ties far behind. The nursing home symbolically embodies the dangerous transition from adulthood to death. It is cut off, clearly bounded, and separated from "normal" life on the "outside." The separation provides artificial safety to the Harrison community, for the isolated residents, tainted as they are by their nearness to death, cannot contaminate others. Douglas described the threat of liminality vividly: "Danger lies in transitional states; simply because transition is neither one state nor the next, it is undefinable. The person who must pass from one to another is himself in danger and emanates danger to others. . . . During the marginal period which separates ritual dying and ritual rebirth, the novices in initiation are temporarily outcast. For the duration of the rite they have no place in society. Sometimes they actually go to live far away outside it. . . . They are not to be blamed for misconduct any more than the foetus in the womb for its spite and greed. . . . It seems that if a person has no place in the social system and is therefore a marginal being, all precaution against danger must come from others. He cannot help his abnormal situation" (1966:116–17). The Harrison community and Franklin staff members put the nursing-home resident into a category distinguishable from themselves as "other." The separation is maintained, continuity is denied, and the apparent danger of contamination thus made remote.

Notebook:
The New Admission

The nurse is talking about Isaac Weitz, the man who died last night. He had lung cancer, but he didn't complain. She sat with him for an hour the day before yesterday because she wanted to give him a chance to say something if he felt like it. She sensed he was going to die soon. Someone says there will be a new admission in two hours. "So soon," says the nurse softly with raised eyebrows. Now she has to make sure that the bed is sanitized and that everything is cleaned up in that room before the new admission arrives and takes the bed.

At 11:00 A.M. the new admission is here, right on schedule. Two social workers are with the man, Hyman Glass, who has been brought by his daughter and son-in-law. "Let's go show Dad his new room," says the social worker brightly, after she introduces Mr. Glass to the nurses. As they go down the hall to Mr. Glass's room, the nurses begin to organize matters for the new admission. One checks his dietary restrictions and calls the kitchen with the information. Another looks through his chart and telephones the physician with a question about medication.

The charge nurse leads the procession to Mr. Glass's new room. He seems affable, is smiling, acts pleased to be introduced to people along the way. At the door, waiting, is Max Sager, Mr. Glass's roommate. Mr. Sager greets Mr. Glass warmly and ceremonially. The charge nurse shows Mr. Glass the various items in the room; she points out where the call light in the bathroom is. Mr. Glass says he doesn't think he will need it, and the charge nurse agrees affably. The daughter comments that her father's problem is that he is too independent.

The social worker notices that there is only one armchair in the

[122]

room and she finds another one in the hall, which she brings in. She comments that this is a nice room because it is at the end of the hall, near the quiet little lounge room. Mr. Sager and Mr. Glass compare notes about what they like to read. The daughter and son-in-law are putting away Mr. Glass's clothing in the bureau drawers. The daughter opens the first drawer and finds toothpaste and a cigarette lighter and seems pleasantly surprised. "Whose are these?" she wants to know. The nurse sees them and quickly snatches them away and with a horrified look on her face, puts them into the trash can.

The social workers ask the daughter and son-in-law to go down-stairs to the social service office in about fifteen minutes, after they have settled her father a little more. When the daughter and son-in-law wait for the elevator to go down, I introduce myself. I ask how the decision was made for Mr. Glass to be admitted, and they say that he is delighted to be here. They repeat that he can be too independent at times. As they go into the elevator, I see a nurse still checking Mr. Glass's records. He is a diabetic, admitted from the hospital. Mr. Glass walks unattended down the hallway a few minutes later. Stan, the orderly, introduces himself genially. Mr. Glass comes over to the nurses' station and talks, and I speak with him. He doesn't remember the name of this place or what it's for. He wants to know if I work here. I explain my research, and he says that he thinks that's nice. A dietician comes to the nurses' station and discusses his food prefer-ences. Mr. Glass asks various people when he will have lunch.

Soon lunch is served in the large dining room. Mr. Glass is shown a table with three other people. They eat wordlessly. After he has fin-ished, he walks over to me. He asks again what the name of the place is. He says he'd been living in Florida and came here to visit. He again wants to know where he is. He asks me about myself and when he hears that I have children, he says, "Well, you know what they say: 'One father can take care of ten children, but ten children can't take care of one father,'" and he smiles.

[7]

Separation and Adaptation: The Passage

Rites of passage are points of crisis within each person's life when certain developmental tasks are faced and changes made. These crises must be resolved successfully so that the individual can proceed smoothly through the life cycle, and the education of the new members can be accomplished. Thus the passages are critical both to those undergoing them and to the group as a whole. As Van Gennep described them they are ordered and predictable, and everyone has a predetermined role in them.

Becoming old in American culture has been considered a rite of passage for which there are few or no rituals (Myerhoff 1982, Keith 1982a), and living in Franklin is comparable to undergoing a symbolic passage from adulthood to death. Separated from their past lives in the community, the residents make adjustment to nursing-home life in various ways described in this and the next chapter. Their lives in the nursing home are liminal: on the threshold, they are stuck in the passage, no longer considered adult, and not yet dead.

The difficulty of the rite of passage, especially liminality, the most dangerous part, makes each person vulnerable, unable to cling to old ways, and emotionally ready to be taught the new ways. As Myerhoff stated:

> Because rites of passage occur at moments of great anxiety, they are dramatic occasions, naturally or socially provided crises, when the person is most teachable. Tension is heightened by rites, and resolution is eagerly sought. The society is then most urgently pressing itself upon the subject of the ceremony, making him or her into its own creature. Yet in the midst of such rituals, individuals are most often aroused to

self-consciousness or brought to the edge of profound questioning by the play with forms—the use of mirrors, masks, costumes, novelty. Borders are crossed; identity symbols stripped away; familiar roles and customs suspended. These conditions make it likely that one may experience that sense of radical privacy, uniqueness, and freedom, the irreversible moment of reflexive awareness, amidst the efforts of the group to impose itself and its interpretations most irresistibly upon the person. Rites of passage invite and forbid independent consciousness at the same moment. (1982:113–15)

Considering all kinds of crises and celebrations as dramaturgical rites of passage, Victor Turner (1967, 1968, 1969, 1974, 1982) included events such as healing ceremonies, protest marches, and carnivals, which, like classic rites of passage, highlight and sometimes reverse normally operating routines of the society. Because everyday cultural rules and behaviors are often turned on their heads during these events, these ritual performances serve as releases from the constraints of the ordinary ways. The positive feelings expressed by anti-war demonstrators of the 1960s and those on religious pilgrimages were some of his examples of communitas. People describe a sense of having shared something extraordinary, of having been in a nether world of mystical-like experience.

Myerhoff (1979) concentrated on crises that arose in the senior center she studied to show how during these times people are thrown back on beliefs that they hold important. These ideas are challenged in the crisis, and if they stand the test, are reasserted with increased validity. The resolution of these problems infuses new life into the beliefs; they are repackaged in new contexts. Their enactment and resolution are like rites of passage, providing continuity for the participants, bringing people together in new ways, and making current old values.

When Goffman stated that "patients start as social infants and end up . . . as resocialized adults" (1961:163) and when he described stripping and mortification procedures that separate an individual from his old role and make him into an inmate, the links to rites of passage are striking. In many rites of passage initiates are made to undergo arduous tasks and must survive physical disfigurement in order to dramatize their bravery and worthiness to enter the new roles.

It would seem that aged Jews who live together in a Jewish nursing home would be able to form a community feeling, but that feeling is lacking in the Franklin Nursing Home. The Jews who enter Franklin

[125]

undergo a rite of passage with important differences. They separate from a past life, but remain heterogeneous and isolated, lacking both ritual support and communitas. With no tasks to perform, they wait.

This chapter describes how individuals begin the rite of passage and make the adjustment to life in the nursing home. It shows how the individual is removed from his former status and station in life and adapts to his new one.

Down in Status

In most rites of passage the person to be initiated proceeds higher in status, usually to the next age grade. The elderly Jew who enters Franklin, however, is demoted in the age-grading system (Goffman 1961:43) by the fact of institutionalization and by what Garfinkle (1956) has referred to as a "degradation ceremony."[1] Becoming old is not everywhere a step down in the world, however. In many societies women and men achieve increased power and prestige when they become very old (see particularly Foner 1984).

When the residents leave behind independent life in the community, dependency is dramatized. Unlike other rites of passage and unlike degradation ceremonies, however, there is no explicit next stage for which admission to the nursing home prepares the entrant.

The Admission Process

The difference between those residents who choose to enter Franklin and those who do not echoes throughout their experiences in the nursing home. People enter the nursing home when they have deficits that cannot be managed on the outside. Thus, a person may manage to avoid institutionalization if he or she lives in a building where architectural design facilitates mobility within the building, where special vans are provided for errands, and where people offer aid. Programs such as Meals on Wheels and daycare facilities also help maintain individuals in their homes. Without these supports, individuals may be unable to function independently and may have to enter a long-term-care facility.

Social and emotional disability can also cripple a person's ability to maintain an autonomous existence. "Why was this person admitted?

Does he have to be here? Could he make it on the outside?" are questions frequently asked by staff members. Often at issue are those persons whose physical disability seems minimal but who manifest disagreeable behaviors. Staff members surmise that these individuals were unable to recruit support from their adult children living nearby because they are unpleasant people.

A precipitating incident often sets the admissions process in motion. A husband and wife hear about a neighborhood robbery, and they begin to ponder the possibility of sheltered care. When an elderly person dies, the spouse is sometimes unable to function. An individual is unable to manage after an illness. Frequently, a number of factors combine to necessitate institutionalization.

Some residents make the decision to enter the nursing home willingly and with understanding of the options available. Charlie Kassin put it this way: "What are you going to do? Thank God. My beautiful daughters each wanted to take me in, but I didn't want them to be jealous of each other. All my life I make good decisions. They expect that of me. They see now I was right. Sure, I'm glad to be here. After my wife died, what else should I do? Lots of these women want me to marry them, but I'm loyal to my wife. I'm glad I decided to come here. The other place was terrible. Here the food is okay; there are things to do; I can do what I want; my kids visit me." However, judging from some of the difficulty Mr. Kassin has had with several residents and staff members, it is possible that his children made it clear that had he asked to live with them, they would have refused.

Ida Kanter expressed no qualms about her decision. She savors her independence, and chuckles about how she determined to be admitted. "After my husband died about thirty years ago, I lived in our house for a while, and then I moved in with my daughter. But she was always after me and worrying about me, and when she worked, she wanted me to look after the dog. After a while I told her I wanted to live by myself. She was upset about what other people would think. 'Who cares what other people think?' I told her, but she worried that everyone would think she was a bad daughter, not taking care of her mother. I got an apartment and lived there while I did volunteer work at the children's center. I'd be there still if I hadn't gotten sick and gone to the hospital. So I decided to come here and recuperate and be with other people. There are things about it I hate, but I'm glad I'm here."

A third resident, Tess Litz, is resigned about her decision to enter the home. She acknowledges her need for it, but she was reluctant to make the move. She never married; she has many brothers and sisters, one of whom is in the nursing home. She broke her hip a year before she was admitted. Everything went "downhill" after the hip fracture. She "wasn't right" afterward. She felt weak, vulnerable, and less capable of functioning on her own. She developed other medical problems, and when there was an opening, she decided to become accustomed to the place before she "really needed it."

These three self-care residents were in a good position to determine their options. The twin ideas of acknowledging need and wishing to maintain autonomy or the semblance of autonomy flow through their narratives. In Mr. Kassin's case, his decision to enter the nursing home may have been a face-saving one, and his situation may be representative of others in the nursing home.

Whether a resident is bitter about admission or not is difficult to know. It is tempting to accept what the resident says about his or her free will in making the decision to come. Visitors, family, and staff do not wish to complicate the situation by probing for signs of discontent, and they accept statements of equanimity when given. Sometimes, however, a resident who seems to be content in the nursing home makes a bitter remark: "Oh sure, we're happy here. The kids pack you up and bring you here, give you a TV, and expect you're all taken care of." On the other hand, it is hard to unravel the statements of residents who sound resentful. Would they be content in their children's homes? Are they bitter about the nursing home, their physical ailments, or their generally decreased physical and social resources? In other cases, the wish to be taken care of may be greater than the need to be taken care of, though the distinction is not a clear-cut one. A staff member expressed her concern to me that some residents give in to dependency too early. For some who saw relatives live their last days at Franklin, the nursing home represents continuity and seems acceptable as a last residence.

Understanding the timing of the entrance into the nursing home is complicated by the fact that the application process may be begun years before the actual admission is made. People may initiate application to the nursing home at the same time that they explore other options, such as living with a son, buying a mobile home, or moving to federally subsidized housing for the elderly. Anticipating an extensive wait and fearing the unpredictability of health, people often begin the application as a hedge against unknown factors arising in the future. When admission is offered to them, their situation is likely to be different; their children may have moved; a daughter may now be divorced and working; the wife's falling spells may have become more frequent. Others seek admission urgently because of dramatic changes in their situation.

Applicants are referred to the nursing home for evaluation via several sources. Typically, a family member or the individual himself makes the initial inquiry. Sometimes, the application is promulgated and completed without the resident's knowledge, though this procedure is discouraged. Social service agencies operating in the community make referrals to the nursing home, as do rabbis and other community leaders. Disposition to the nursing home is increasingly often made from the hospital during an acute illness for which continuing care is required. An interview and other procedures are conducted with the social service staff. Information pertaining to the individual's financial and health status are necessary, and this information is checked against other sources of information.[2] After the application has been made and the social worker has written an evaluation, the case comes before a meeting of the admissions committee. Members of the committee try to gauge the immediacy and the severity of need, and they determine whether admission will be granted to the individual. When the decision is affirmative, the person is apprised of the approximate time until admission.

Social workers have noted that the decision to enter the nursing home is often traumatic. They relate anecdotes about how some applicants "give up" after they acknowledge that they must be admitted. They consider some of the individuals who die between the time of the application and the actual admission to be cases of "hidden suicide." One said: "I haven't kept actual count, but I'd swear that in the last year, at least three people who have gone through the entire admission process, and have then been told that it's time to be admitted, have then either died just before their admission day, or right after. Maybe the blow of having to come in here, of knowing that one cannot make it on the outside, does it to them."

Usually a bed becomes available because of death. It is rare that an individual leaves this nursing home, though there have been instances of this happening over the years. When a death occurs, the person who is next in line is usually admitted within the week. For some people it is a relief to enter the nursing home and have the security that it represents. For example, Gerald Wiedenbaum credits his admission for saving his life:

Mr. Wiedenbaum had a satisfying life until a few years prior to admission when things began to unravel for him. His wife developed Alzheimer's disease. In the beginning her behavior was confusing and frightening because they did not know what was happening. At the same time, Mr. Wiedenbaum's successful light-fixture business was proving to be too much work. He sold his store. The family physician urged him to take a vacation in Florida and to initiate the admission process to the Franklin Nursing Home for both of them. When they were admitted, he was relieved. He was a "nervous wreck" and in terrible health from worry over his wife and the strenuous caretaking of her that was becoming increasingly necessary.

For other residents admission is instead a recognition that the end is near, and there are no alternatives. Few people who enter the home are misled about their being there, but for those who are, the adjustment can be more difficult (see below).

Admission day is a big transition. Usually the resident has already visited the nursing home. On the day of admission, he is typically accompanied by one or more members of his family. There are paperwork, introductions, and unpacking. The actual admission is accomplished privately between the new resident, the social worker, and a family member or friend. As the new admission is introduced to staff members and residents who live on the floor, the major adjustment to life in the nursing home begins.

The First Three Months

The first six weeks to three months are considered by the staff to be a vulnerable time for the new resident. This vulnerability is reflected in the mortality rate, which is high in the first thirty days and levels off over the next few months (Clinton, Shield, and Aronson 1983). It is unclear whether the mortality rate is high because many residents enter with fundamentally terminal illness or whether other factors, such as stress attending the transition, are involved.

Staff members have noted that when a newly admitted resident refers to the nursing home as "home," a milestone has been reached, and adjustment to the nursing home has been made. In contrast, Laird (1979) recalled how afraid she was of lapsing into the habit of calling the nursing home "home." She equated this usage with succumbing to the torpor of accepting her lot within the nursing home and resisted the temptation strenuously.

To some, entering the nursing home means giving up the outside and autonomous living in the community. Others refuse such meanings. They adjust to the nursing home pragmatically: they accept the added safeguards and security that the nursing home provides, and they negotiate their way through the system, picking and choosing among activities and people. Marjorie Tempkin is an example.

She was admitted only seven weeks ago and is adjusting remarkably well to life on the self-care unit. She is 80 years old, was born in Poland, married at 20, has been widowed for many years, and never had children. She was a teacher at an elementary school until retiring in the late 1960s. Only one brother remains alive. She expresses satisfaction with her career as a teacher. Mrs. Tempkin was admitted because of falling spells, heart illness, and diabetes. She has kept her subscriptions to theater and chamber music series, and she goes to these events with old friends. She expresses disbelief that few of the other residents are interested in attending these performances. One of the things she insisted on bringing into the nursing home was her stereo record player and record collection. She has adapted her room to suit her needs; for example, the tray that goes over the bed works well as a letter-writing table. Her phone rings often as various nieces and friends inquire how she is doing. Relieved to be here, she feels secure that should she fall or have heart trouble, the nursing home is equipped to deal with these problems. She just wishes the weekends were not so very long and boring. It is difficult to get through them.

Therefore, many residents improve after admission. They may have been undernourished, depressed, lonely, and in bad physical health and, following admission to the nursing home, may become better. They are happy to have other people around them; they like the food; they are pleased to join activities. Many residents have an expanded social sphere after entering the nursing home. For example, a woman who was previously afraid to leave her apartment is now able to play bingo, have regular exercise, and be helped in needlework. Perhaps

[131]

for the first time in years she is persuaded to vote in a federal election.[3]

On the other hand, residents who do not know that the move to the nursing home is intended to be permanent have more difficulty in adjusting than do those who know and have prepared for the move with this knowledge.

Mrs. Grosz's son feels that in his mother's eyes, he is the worst son. Furthermore, because he has had a difficult relationship with her all his life, he does not want to incur her wrath by telling her the truth. He does not want the responsibility of taking care of her in his home. Since entering the nursing home, she has been eating better and getting stronger. She now wants to go home, and refuses to participate in any of the activities. She has not been told that her son has released the apartment.

Though the staff members expressed their disapproval of Mrs. Grosz's family for not telling her the truth, they also thought that a person like Mrs. Grosz would be a difficult addition to a household. They both sympathized with the family's predicament and were critical of the deception that was perpetrated.

Giving up the Outside

The move to the nursing home is physically and emotionally arduous. "Breaking up" the apartment is the term used to describe the procedure of deciding which items to take to the nursing home and how the other items are to be disposed of. As Gubrium writes: "Breaking up a home means losing ties with many people, objects, and places. Most recall the loss of loved ones—a spouse, children, a friend—with whom they once made a home. Their histories store memories of birthdays, weddings, and other times when someone, now gone, was somehow linked to them. . . . As clientele speak of objects, the things seem to come alive. Breaking ties with objects blurs a set of sentiments as does breaking ties with people. . . . The familiar trivia of everyday life are often the hallmarks of solid ties. The presence of trivial items, easily noticeable, assures one that, indeed, all is basically 'as usual' in one's life. The long-term absence of familiar trivia is alarming, for it signals change" (1975:86–87). Depending on whether the individual enters the wing or the new building, the new resident has some choice about what items—such as rugs, blankets, knickknacks, ornaments, and mementos—may be imported from the outside. Deciding what items to choose becomes a matter of determining which ones contain the highest concentration of practical and emotional significance and fit the requirements of the nursing home and the available space.[4] All at once the one room (or half a room) in the nursing home becomes bedroom and living room together.

Mrs. Zeldin didn't want to give up many of her possessions when she came here. What was she to pick? This little table had some memories attached to it, and she could use it in her new room, and it was the right size, so it came with her. But she really liked the way her dining room and bedroom had been set up. Giving pieces away was hard, too: Her niece would never truly appreciate them, never understand their true significance.

For residents who are capable and who know their circumstances with precise clarity, the reduction in things and the limitation of access to things is made worse by the symbolic significance that attaches to those things.

It is taking a lot out of Tess Litz to keep going back and forth to her apartment, deciding what to keep, what to give away, and what to throw away. She is anxious to have this job over, and she is grateful to the patient social worker who is putting up with her slow decision-making process. Miss Litz keeps telling herself that things will be better once all these possessions have been gone through and she then begins to settle in here. On her lap right now is a box jammed with letters that she is looking over, one by one. Which ones should she keep?

Mrs. Safrin talked about a favorite doll that she wished she had never given away because it summed up and made tangible the positive memories she had of her childhood, which, in many ways, had been a hard one. Not having the doll in her present circumstances makes her feel that the past in which the doll was present did not truly exist. Residents may miss the kitchen table where meals were shared; they

[133]

miss the furniture carefully saved for and chosen and polished through the years. The items were clues to those memories now in doubt because of the things' absence.

An individual must relinquish a number of other things in order to be admitted. One is his or her driver's license. Most residents are too sick to drive.[5] The feeling of loss surrounding not being able to drive remains among some residents. Sarah Zeldin said simply, "You may as well be dead if you don't have your car." She resents having to make special arrangements in order to go out. She bristles at reminders of her dependency on others. It is difficult for her to reciprocate the rides that others give her since she thinks there are no favors she can offer in return. Stanley Fierstein is bitter that he cannot drive. Though he made the decision to enter the nursing home, he seems to blame the nursing home for his restricted activities. He conceptualizes his loss as a reduction in both autonomy and privacy. He would like, for example, to take a friend to a movie or to a restaurant whenever he feels like it, and without everyone else knowing about it. The cluster of meanings that automobiles have for American adults probably does not disappear with old age.

Another significant loss is one's former home and address. The resident who owned a home or condominium usually had to sell it in order to pay the expenses of the nursing home. This decision can be a bitter one. The resident usually cannot retain inheritable property and still pay for long-term care. The other ignominious alternative is to divest all assets and become eligible for Medicaid. Though most residents have had to use Medicaid assistance, there is considerable stigma attached.[6]

More losses from the previous environment (not including the hospital) are the refrigerator, favorite chairs and furniture, a garden, separate rooms, and the space and privacy that accompany these items. Many residents experience the loss of their refrigerators keenly. A resident who wants something to eat or drink must either request it from a staff member or wait until the next meal. Though it is possible to buy something on the outside and store it in the communal refrigerator on the floor, space in the refrigerator is limited, and the food is likely to be eaten by someone else. Residents can offer little to a guest. For most of the women this inability to give a guest something to eat is difficult. Usually they keep a glass jar filled with hard candies for this purpose. I was often "rewarded" for my visits by having candy or other treats pressed on me.

Food means more than its immediate functional characteristics. Food is basic to nurturing and being taken care of. Smells, tastes, and textures of food remind people of their childhoods, of their mothers, of their children, of being loved by adults.

Sarah Zeldin was saying, "Today when I woke up, I had the most incredible desire to stir a cake."

Food has added associations for women who link it with their roles as mothers and to their past and present relationships with their children. Food often defines women as women: how well they nourish their children, how competently they entertain guests.

Marjorie Tempkin says that one of the things she thinks she is going to miss the most about living here is that she won't be able to provide meals to her friends. Though she'll keep up many of the activities that she enjoyed doing with them, it's going to be hard not to be able to invite them home for something homemade to eat.

Giving up space, personal possessions, and means of mobility have the result of limiting the physical sphere in which the individual functions. Individuals who are easily confused may fare well when choices are restricted and space limited. The hospital-like routines lend a predictable regularity to the victim of Alzheimer's disease, whose memory is failing, whose judgment is haphazard, whose physical abilities to tend himself have deteriorated. Old things, routines, associations, and statuses are given up when residents enter the nursing home. But the process of adaptation involves not merely adjustment to a series of losses. Concomitant with relinquishing possessions and routines of the life lived outside the institution is the acclimatization to patterns and routines inside the institution.

Taking on the Inside

The new resident receives an identification wristband and learns the physical layout of the room to which he is assigned as well as the building and grounds. He is subjected to new sights, sounds, and smells that may be unwelcome and frightening and which are difficult to avoid. Loudspeakers in all the hallways are used to call staff members to meetings, alert them to telephone calls, dictate to the residents what day it is, and itemize the activities that are about to begin. The sounds of demented residents penetrate far down the hallways. Some of the sounds are moans, some are cries for help, others are beseeching a long dead mother, others are screams about unknown (to others) terrors. Some of the residents emit wheezing, coughing, choking, and spitting sounds, depending on their physical condition. Adapting to these sounds is difficult, but most residents eventually are able to screen them out.

While listening to Bernice Meyerhov, I was distracted by the screeching "help" cry I heard from somewhere down the hall. Finally, I asked Mrs. Meyerhov what it was. "Oh," she replied simply, "that's just Mr. Wolf. He's meshuga [crazy] and does that all the time."

Successful acclimatization to the nursing home probably involves the ability to tune out unwanted stimuli of all sorts. Neglecting to turn on one's hearing aid has this adaptive function.

Smells are numerous, as well. The smells of the food trucks coming down the halls are usually welcome ones. Other smells are those of urine, feces, and, much more often, disinfectants and other harsh cleaning fluids in use all the time.[7]

Mrs. Price and I have just come up the elevator to the second floor and are now walking past the nurses' station to her room located nearby. The smell of ammonia is strong. "I just can't get used to that smell," comments Mrs. Price.

New residents must also witness sights that are disturbing. Some of the sickest residents are kept near the nurses' station where they can be watched easily. Being central and public may be as uncomfortable for the watched resident as it is for the others. Occasionally, too, residents may find themselves unwillingly witnessing other residents who are naked.

Mrs. Zeldin told me that the nursing assistant once left the door open while she was putting a diaper on her neighbor. The neighbor had her back to the hallway and was leaning against the chest of drawers while the nursing assistant was putting the diaper on her. Mrs. Zeldin was horrified and ashamed for her neighbor, though she understood that her neighbor probably did not care since she was not "all there." "I keep thinking: what if that happens to me?" said Mrs. Zeldin.

Sometimes, during evenings, nights, and on weekends, staff members undress residents in their rooms and take them down the corridors for bathing. These behaviors are not allowed by the administration, but they sometimes occur during off-hours when shifts are understaffed and supervisors are not present.

Family members often buy something for the new resident's room, such as a television, a fan, a small piece of furniture, or something functional. Gerald Wiedenbaum's family, for instance, bought him a portable closet because they wanted him to be able to continue his practice of collecting good clothes and dressing well. On the other hand, when Mrs. Safrin's family bought her a television set, she thought they were washing their hands of her.

The strategies residents learn are numerous and varied. They learn to categorize other residents, to differentiate among the staff, and they learn the staff hierarchies. These distinctions enable them to know how and to whom to register complaints and to devise techniques to have their needs and wants fulfilled. Orientation to the way the nursing home operates is made quite rapidly by the residents. Residents learn about activities and services; they know the nursing shifts, the not-nice from the nice personnel; they learn which staff members will be available for favors and which will not be.

One of the most important distinctions capable residents learn to make is between the people who are mentally competent and those who are not. Generally, those residents who are in the wing consider the residents "over there" or "on the other side" to be sick and senile. They maintain as much physical and psychological distance as possible from these people.

Living in close quarters among a heterogeneous group of people with whom one does not choose to be, one must devise ways of controlling and avoiding those one dislikes. Residents who are the most physically and intellectually able usually desire to surround themselves with people whom they like. Generally, they do not wish to be exposed to those residents who are either very ill or have "lost their marbles." Probably the most common mechanism that residents use to limit their contact with the confused residents is to ignore them. Pretending that they do not exist, the alert residents can shield themselves quite effectively from verbal contact with them.

[137]

Mr. Rosen did not know that Mrs. Simonson was crazy at first. She had just been admitted and she was assigned to the dining table in a seat directly opposite his. During the first meal he said that he tried to act like a gentleman, and he asked her a little about herself. Immediately she accused him of taking her food and started to yell. Finally, Mr. Rosen said with righteous anger, "Madame, you have finished your meal; I have not yet started mine. Will you please allow me to eat and leave me alone?" He stated with satisfaction that his pronouncement startled and quieted her. Now he ignores her, knowing that if he even looks at her, she will start something.

The primary mealtime strategy is avoidance. Because there is opportunity for argument and misunderstanding when people talk, the alert residents usually stay relatively silent.

Mrs. Zeldin said that if she wants to talk to Mrs. Kanter, she never does so at the dinner table. She waits until they are together in one of their rooms by themselves. After all, if she says something to Mrs. Kanter at the table, the crazy ones interrupt, want to know what they're talking about, and garble what is being said. It's aggravating and not worth it. So they keep quiet during dinner.

It is hard to avoid the confused residents, even on the self-care unit. They may live across the hall or next door, and they intrude themselves on the more competent residents. Sometimes they will not tolerate evasive treatment and become insistent. These residents have to be treated differently.

Mrs. Gottschalk lives across the hall from Frannie Kerman. She is anxious and confused. She asks the same questions day and night. Her behavior irritates Mrs. Gottschalk and often upsets her. But Mrs. Kerman cannot be avoided. Mrs. Gottschalk has finally adapted to Mrs. Kerman's incessant questioning in a formulaic and detached way. Now when the lunch truck comes by, Mrs. Gottschalk calls out, "Frannie, it's time to eat now. You can leave your pocketbook in your room. Call your daughter after." In this way she anticipates the flurry of questions that are predictable each and every mealtime.

For self-protection, many residents keep to themselves. Wary of involvements—positive attachments and dependencies as well as negative interactions—many of the residents consider it a virtue "not to bother anyone" and to "behave" oneself. A bland, superficial interaction style is characteristic of the relationships that evolve within the nursing home as a result. This subject will be dealt with at greater length in a subsequent chapter.

Socializing to the nursing home seems to be aided by other residents and by certain staff, such as a sympathetic nursing assistant, orderly, nurse, or social worker. Who socializes whom is also dependent upon the neediness of the resident, his desires to be helped, and his personality. A resident who steadfastly refuses to socialize with others will be urged only so much to do so. As a staff member said: "Mrs. Grosz stays in her room most of the day and seems angry when asked to join us at activities. Most of the other residents are staying away from her as well. We think it would be helpful if she could be persuaded to come to activities, but at least right now, she really doesn't want to. She's mean to everyone." Therefore, residents and staff members often let a resident who wishes to remain by herself stay by herself.

Residents learn, furthermore, the constraints of the system. They know the rules by which the organization works. They learn to accept that their food preferences cannot be fulfilled for budgetary reasons, for example, or that a food mix-up may result from the fact that mistakes often happen in a hierarchical organization: "One of the supreme pleasures of my day," Mrs. Zeldin is telling me, "is to have my tomato juice with my meal. I am allowed to have salted tomato juice, but every now and then, they either don't have it, or they give me the unsalted by mistake. Only when it's their mistake, they refuse to believe it. What are you going to do about that? Make sure that they hire college graduates who know the difference between tomato juices?" While recognizing that it is foolish to battle too many issues in the nursing home because the chances of success are minimal, residents also learn how to gather important information regarding staff, for example. One resident decided that a social worker was not working there anymore because her name was no longer called over the loudspeaker. Residents piece together information from various sources: one resident may have a good relationship with a particular aide; another always chats with the janitor. The ties and contacts are intricate and go outside the institution, as Gubrium (1975) has also noted. Thus, one resident may have been a teacher to the social worker twenty years before, and the social worker's mother frequents

[139]

the resident's sister's fabric shop. The transmission of information takes place in all these ways.

Entering the nursing home is a rite of passage with important differences from most rites of passage. As in all rites of passage, the participants dramatically leave things and associations that accompanied them in their former status. Entering the nursing home is a concrete sign that autonomous living in the community is impossible. The new resident must become accustomed to new things such as rules, sights, sounds, and new people. Some of the procedures by which an old person becomes a nursing-home resident are formal and routinized, much as they might be in other rites of passage. But unlike in other rites of passage, the individual leaves his former station and enters a new realm largely unaccompanied by others. There is no welcoming ceremony or newcomers' club; there is nothing public about the admissions process. Instead, it is carried out between the social worker, the resident and a family member, and perhaps the nurse on the resident's floor. There are no gifts, nor are there announcements. Entrance to the nursing home is a momentous occasion, but a private and solitary one.

Notebook:
The Kitchen

Today I have arranged to be with Bess Klein, a dietician. I go to the office downstairs to wait for her. Everything is in an uproar these days. The cook of eleven years has been fired, and there have been various cooks since. One is in the hospital. An older man was just fired because he was too nervous to stand the chaos of the kitchen. One of the cooking assistants is smoking and making cracks. The dietary assistant tells him that he shouldn't smoke, but he continues.

Bess comes in. She says she was going to cancel me a million times but then she decided that it's always this way, so "what the heck." She stuffs her pocketbook in the second drawer of the file cabinet and advises me to do the same. She hands me a hairnet, and we both put them on. One of the staff comes in and tells Bess that they had to return a delivery of Campbell soups because they weren't kosher. Someone ordered them wrong.

Bess instructs me: Because institutional foods start looking and tasting the same after a while, she breaks up the pattern by having different things each week, with the beginning of the menu cycle occurring every four weeks. The cycle is further varied by holiday meals, luncheons (where people can cheat on their diets), parties, and so forth. She takes into account the variety, color, texture, and flavor of food in devising menus. There's also a spring menu, a fall menu, and so forth. Supper is the dairy meal, which is good, since the elderly need a lighter meal at the end of the day. The main meal is at lunchtime. The exception is on Friday nights, Shabbos, when roast chicken is always served. Most residents love chicken and would prefer to have it always. On Saturday lunch they have chicken again; cold soups, fruit, and cottage cheese are typical Saturday-evening fare because cooking is prohibited on the Sabbath. Now it's Succos, so there are traditional foods like honeycake on the menu.

Breakfasts are the same each week. The state mandates the size of portions and stipulates how much protein and other nutritional quantities should be included. Therefore such figurings and other dietary requirements are added to the voluminous paperwork that the state sees during inspections.

Bess takes me through the kitchen. She asks a few of the staff how various residents are eating. A woman who would eat only in the evening seems to be doing a little better. Her devoted nursing assistant had noticed that if she was given Robitussin a half-hour before her meals she would cough up mucus and be able to eat. Other staff members had merely commented that the woman was too congested to eat. Bess is exasperated by such cursory reports on residents, against which the observations of a caring nursing assistant stand out so prominently. In this case Bess blames the fourth-floor charge nurse, who is usually watching television. "You get to know who the better nurses are," comments Bess.

She says that people need to be encouraged to eat properly. It is psychologically better for a person to eat regular food than blended food. Brisket and hamburger and steak all look alike when they are blended; so do cauliflower and rice and noodles. Many people need help with their food, but don't always get it. When the kitchen sends oranges on the trays they are often returned untouched; presumably staff workers haven't bothered to peel them.

Bess shows me huge sinks filled with steaming water kept at 180 degrees for pots and pans. The dairy side of the kitchen adjoins the meat side. There are different sets of silverware and pots and dishes to conform to kosher laws. Everything is prepared the day before. Juices are portioned out and kept in the refrigerator. Whatever can be done earlier is done earlier. Some men are emptying the dishwasher. Bess looks over the silverware that has just been cleaned. Dairy ware has accidentally been mixed with the meat ware. This sometimes happens when a few stray pieces from the night before get put into the dishwasher with the morning dishes. Though they try to keep everything separate, such things can't be helped.

While we are touring the kitchen in this way, various employees are asking her questions: "Mrs. K., where are the orange cards?" "Mrs. K., I took fifteen minutes less yesterday so I want to leave fifteen minutes early today." "Mrs. K., the noise on the dishwasher stopped and it won't work." She looks at me and says that she has to be a mechanic, too. Somehow she fixes it. The person looking for the orange cards returns, unsuccessful in his search. Bess goes to the storage room, where we rummage for fifteen minutes through the cases of soups, cookies, and huge kitchen utensils that are piled everywhere. No orange cards. As we come out of the storage room, today's cook wants to know if extra help can be called in since they're short staffed today. Bess doesn't think so and says that these are bad times. The cook raises his eyes heavenward; Bess takes off to do something else.

Soon we go back to the dairy kitchen. She shows me the elaborate card file setup. There is a separate card file for each floor, and each resident has an alphabetized card in the file. The card indicates the person's diet and has space for changes through time. Also listed are preferences and dislikes for each meal. "This is our Bible, and things go well when it's completely followed and updated," says Bess. Today, for example they are making blintzes for lunch. Looking at the files, one can see at a glance that some people like doubles, and some people don't like blintzes at all. Substitutions are available too.

The trays are set up like this: in an assembly-line fashion, one person puts the silverware, napkin, salt, saccharin, tea, Sanka, and other dry things on the tray according to the preferences on the card file. When the tray advances to the hot food, another person reads from the file. "Silver doesn't like squash; give her the noodles, but no sour cream, extras on the blintzes, but no plums." While the half-dozen or so people who are doing this are working, Bess is adding things, checking, correcting mistakes. She or one of the others supervises the line each meal. Depending on the needs of the residents, there are blended foods and superblends and no-salt varieties. Half-trays for hot foods and half-trays for cold foods are assembled together onto the proper shelf of the food truck by each resident's name, which is marked on both sides of the shelf. Nurses on the floors reassemble the trays in the proper order for each resident. Nonetheless, mistakes happen frequently.

After each food truck is filled, the jobs are rotated. This procedure ensures that the system isn't dependent on any particular person and everyone learns every job. One by one the individual food trucks are loaded and sent out of the kitchen. Bess notices that one of the trucks has something loose on it, and she makes a note on her pad to have it fixed. We go out into the hall where the trucks are to make sure they

[143]

are heating up properly. Finding two that aren't, Bess says, "I tell them every day to make sure all the right lights are on, but I'm not dealing with college graduates here. My staff is good, but things like this happen all the time." She yells at Fernando and tells him to send the cold food truck out last so that it has a chance to heat up.

Years back, there were pieces of paper stuck everywhere indicating the no-added salt, the no-lactose, the extra blintzes, the doubles on custards—all the preferences, dislikes, and therapeutic diets that are on the card file now. When Bess first began, she went with pad in hand to every floor and asked each resident what he or she wanted for dinner and for supper the next day. But too much time was spent hearing about the son who wasn't visiting or the shoulder that destroyed last night's sleep or the nurse who was grumpy, and furthermore, when mealtime came and the resident would look to see what his or her neighbor had, he would decide that he liked the other meal better than his own, or he might forget that he had ordered what he had ordered. It was much too difficult a system to manage. Thus began the four-week cycle of meal plans. The menus are posted on each floor in accordance with state law, and everyone gets the same menu with the preferences and dislikes individualizing the system. However, the nurses always lose track of which week of the cycle it is, so no one knows which meal is next.

On the meat side of the kitchen, a woman is taking apart boiled chickens that were used for the chicken soup. She is putting the breasts neatly on a pan and removing the bones. "Some people would prefer to have boiled chicken every day," says Bess, "but we can't do that." She and the woman talk about what to do with the brisket that just came out of the oven and what she can cook ahead. Because the stuffed cabbage is frozen, her work is a little easier today.

The cook approaches and insists that they are really short: couldn't she please call in someone else. Without looking at him, she says, "Okay, when you're right, you're right"; surprised, he shrugs his shoulders, and leaves. She makes two phone calls for replacements: the first person isn't in, and she leaves a message for the second.

Bess tells me, "Another problem for the elderly people, you know, is that with all the other things that go, taste goes too. People put sugar in their soup, in so many things, just to give flavor." While she's speaking, she sees a man come in and greet her. "Oh no," she groans, and goes to speak to him. This is the man who was fired because he was too flustered in the kitchen. Bess had given the message to his *daughter, but it obviously had not got through. Now she is telling him that although he is very nice, he made some mistakes, didn't get some amounts right, doesn't seem to have enough experience, and how sorry she is. He's nodding and smiling and agreeing. He wants to know if he can go back on Social Security, and Bess refers him to the budget department upstairs. "I nearly died when I saw him," she says to me when he leaves.*

The cook wants to know where the tomato sauces are for the lasagna. They have to make both the salt-free and the regular. They find a whole vat of regular sauce already prepared in the refrigerator and can't figure out why it's there. It must be that last night's cook mistakenly thought she was supposed to make it. In any case, it comes in handy now! Also, it is discovered that everyone received the regular sauce last time it was served. Oops.

Bess has me look over the spiral notebook that contains patient-care policies: goals of the food service, mechanisms of the therapeutic diets, sizes of portions, where the menus are posted, and job descriptions for all the kitchen jobs. While I'm looking at these items, Bess orders chickens—she had asked three people, including me, to remind her to do this—and other foods over the phone too. She hands me a piece of paper. It is a form filled out by a nurse, which indicates that a particular resident is going to have a lab procedure and will therefore be restricted to a liquid diet for tomorrow's meals. "This is the only nurse who ever lets me know when there's something like this. She's the only one who informs me the proper way. They never do it. They either call me at the last moment, or they don't bother to inform me at all."

Bess phones someone else. "Did the ad get in the paper? Thank God! Okay, goodbye." She turns to me. No one wants to work anymore. It's amazing, considering the economy these days (the 10.1 percent unemployment figure just came out today). It used to be that when she'd place an ad, scores of people would respond: women who said they could cook because they'd fed their families for so many years, and others with experience and without. With this ad, she has received only three responses, and it has run from Wednesday through Sunday. One man sounded good and supposedly had twenty years of experience, but he couldn't document any of the places where he'd worked. . . .

Someone tells Bess that there is a terrible smell of gas in the kitchen and "all the girls are complaining about it." Bess leaves to investigate. When we return to the kitchen we find that many of the trucks have been sent up to the floors. So it's a mad dash to run up to the floors to check out residents' reactions to the meal. First we go to the second-floor dining room. Bess goes around to the residents, admonishing them to eat more, taking complaints, and writing down changes. She asks the nursing assistants how so-and-so is doing, and one nursing assistant says that this resident loves this custard and should get more. Bess writes it down. One resident tells Bess that she's always mistaken for another resident and she doesn't like it. Bess sympathizes. Hyman Glass is reminded not to take ice cream from the trays of other residents. "You're not supposed to eat ice cream, Mr. Glass." "I can eat anything!" he retorts. "I know you can, but your doctor says you can't, so I'm not allowed to give it to you!" Bess answers expertly.

Now we go to the nurses' station to tell the nurses to watch Mr. Glass's ice-cream-stealing ways. We run up the stairs to the third floor and make the rounds of the residents. Some of the nursing assistants are feeding various residents. One man is coughing very badly. A woman is leaving the dining room, saying that she has no appetite around these old people who sound so bad. Bess suggests to a nurse that this resident eat in her room for a few days. This seems to be arranged. Another resident tells Bess that she doesn't like the food. Bess says that since she's only been here one day, she will get used to it. The resident replies that she's been here a week. Bess persists that it's been one day until a nursing assistant verifies that the resident has been here a week. Bess apologizes.

Suddenly, one woman yells, "I have to go to the bathroom!" A few staff people pass her without looking. We go by a table where the residents have already left their seats. A pill lies serenely in a paper cup, which prompts Bess to mutter, "I thought they were supposed to watch patients taking meds." Now she checks some of the trays that have been left by the residents. We see that cups of coffee were poured in several cases, and that the tea bag or the packet of Sanka on the tray was left unopened. "You see," says Bess, with bitterness, "we try to individualize things, but they go and pour everyone coffee, never stopping to notice the Sanka or the tea bag. What can you do?"

Now, quick up to the fourth floor. One of the orderlies tell us that a particular resident is doing great on this floor. Bess scoffs to me, "Sure, he wasn't doing well on the second floor, but he does well here," meaning that he is receiving different, that is, better, care here. Now we check trays put back in the truck, ask about residents who

*didn't eat well or who are out (but Bess hadn't been notified again),
note the unopened Sanka packets and the dry tea bags, coax people to
try things. Lo and behold, some of them do try the food when they are
urged.*

*Up to the fifth floor. Bernice Meyerhov is hovering over her broth-
er. Bess comes over and says that she's wonderful to her brother,
helping him eat, but meanwhile she has eaten nothing herself. Mrs.
Meyerhov smiles impishly and shrugs her shoulders, saying the food
doesn't appeal to her; she doesn't want to force herself. Bess urges
someone else to eat more, but this resident says no, it's too much, she's
had enough. Other residents call her over—to request something different; to ask for more soup; to remind Bess that she hates plums. Bess
writes it all down.*

*Now, hurry, over to the third-floor wing. As we approach the din-
ing area, Bess warns me that she expects many complaints here. She
calls, "Is it safe to come in here?" and the nurse calls back, "No!" but
we continue. Sarah Zeldin reproaches me for not having seen her for a
week. Ida Kanter asks Bess why the kitchen couldn't spare her two
slices of cheese. Mrs. Zeldin wants to know why she didn't get tomato
juice, and she doesn't want to eat the blintzes; she whispers to me that
they're "lousy and tough." Mrs. Zeldin asks me, "What's eating her
today?" and then asks Bess, "Can you get me an Abie Abramson so I
can get my food earlier?" and Bess retorts, "You need an Abie, that's
for sure." Mrs. Zeldin says they run out of food by the time the last
trays are given out. As we leave, Bess remembers why there's no
tomato juice for Mrs. Zeldin: no one got any today because they didn't
have any today. The nurse, allying with Bess, calls out sarcastically,
"Well, that's no excuse."*

*Down to the second floor of the wing. Bess explains to Stanley
Fierstein that a favorite food that he has been requesting is too expensive to purchase right now. She tells him that when the price comes
down a little, they will get it. A nurse whispers rather loudly to me and
to Bess, "I know what it is: they think it's a hotel. They're spoiled."
Bess tells me that one problem is that the residents on the wing are
allowed more choices in their meals, but they forget what it was they
chose. "I don't know if it's worth all the trouble and the aggravation,"
says Bess.*

*We go downstairs to the kitchen. Bess is tired. It is frustrating
work. She takes out her notebook and reviews some of her observa-*

tions with some of her staff: why this went wrong, why this substitu-tion wasn't made, and so on. One employee is peeling potatoes; then someone else finds out that a whole pot of peeled potatoes is already in the refrigerator, waiting to be cooked. Bess has been here very late the last few nights: 10:30 last night, 1:00 A.M. a few nights before. She doesn't know how late she'll be here tonight.

Voice: Ida Kanter

I am 94 years old, born and raised on a farm. My sisters and brothers were all born there, and we had a wonderful time. My folks sent for their parents from Russia, and when they came in, there was no room for them to sleep. We had chicken coops, and we had to take all the chickens out and put them in the woods so there would be a place to sleep in. There was room for them to eat in the house—one set—then at another time another set would come in. And that's the way it was until we got a little older, and we had to go to grammar school. It was a little bit too far, and the snow was way up—so my parents decided we had to move. So we moved to another part of the city, and we lived there for quite a while. And I met my husband there. But before that I worked at the department store. I had only been working I guess it was three weeks when the High Holidays— Rosh Hashanah—came along. And I asked to go out, and [the supervisor] said, "You only just come in and you want to go out. What's the big idea?" I says, "It's a holiday." He says, "Holiday? What kind of a holiday now?" I says, "New Year's." "New Year's? In September? What's the big idea?" I said, "I happen to be Jewish." "I thought you were Polish." My name was Kosinsky. So he says, "You prefer your religion to working here?" "Well," I says, "I like my religion." "Stay home!" So I went to get my things, and he said, "You can work a couple of days more and that's it!" I came home and I cried. I said, "I got such a good job," and I didn't like the idea of the holidays coming in. And my mother and father said, "Well, God will be good to you." Monday morning I got up, and where was I going to go? The only place that would take Jewish people would be Hiller's Department

Store. And I had a whole book of stamps to go on the trains—it cost me five dollars, and I had just got it. So I thought I'd try it. As I was getting ready to take the 11:17 train, the telephone bell rang. "Miss Kosinsky?" I said yes. The secretary said, "Just a minute." He said, "Why'n't you come to work?" "You told me to stay home!" "Take the next train." I said, "I'm waiting for it now." He said, "See that you're on it." Well, anyway, I worked there for ten years. After that he was just like a father to me. I was only 17, 18, 19. He'd watch me just like a father would watch. Anything he would want to know about the Jewish religion, he would ask me. He was really a very very nice man.

My father was a very religious man. My mother was very religious. I kept the faith, and after I was married I kept a kosher house. I guess I was the only one. When I got married, I got in-laws and outlaws. My husband's aunt and uncle came over here, and then she died and I was left with the old man. He was with me for fifteen years. And that's the way it was—until my husband died. Of course my daughters were big. There were grandchildren—there they are up there [points to a photograph on the wall]. When he passed away I went to live with one daughter, Ethel. I was in my seventies. She was working, now she's retired—sales manager. She left me with the dog. He'd walk with me a couple of steps, then run ahead. So I said to Ethel one day, "I got to go back." I'd broken up my house—eight rooms—but I took an apartment. And so it was until I was 89 and I went back to live with my daughter and the dog. And I would sit on the porch—my daughter would be at work—and I'd see an airplane and I'd say to Jack, the dog, "Look at the airplane," and he'd look at me. And I said to Ethel, "I'm going into the home." She looked like she'd been shot. I said it'll be better for me, and it'll be better for you. So they brought me in. They showed me a room, and I looked out the window and I saw kids out there and a garden and I made friends with them through the window, and I said to them, "This is the room I'm going to have." Four years, this room.

When I came in the first time, no one spoke to me. Except Phyllis the nurse, she was very nice to me. We had a very nice group of people, but they all died out. Six people died in one year. I could make friends very easily.

So I sit here and I read. I just started this one. Very bold, very sassy girl—very sassy. There's a wealthy man and the girl wants to run away from her mother, and the man hasn't decided who to give the

*money to. This is my library—want to borrow some books? All the
nurses come in. I've about fifteen or twenty [romance] books out.
Here, take one. This is cute; take this one.*

*When I was a girl we had a cow, we had six geese and a gander, and
we had chickens. We did all our own planting, and we had two big
chestnut trees right in the middle of the orchard. We had all kinds of
vegetables, all kinds of fruits. Some of the kids used to come by and
break down the limbs, and I used to sit with a stick and say, "If you
want some fruit, I will give you some. But if you break the limbs, next
year when you come back, there won't be any fruit." I used to walk
around with the stick. My father made a great big stone wall [root
cellar] where he used to store all the things: the carrots, the cabbage,
the string beans, everything, so in the wintertime, we'd open up this
great big wall and go in and get the things that we wanted. The apples,
the potatoes, the beets, the carrots, everything—sometimes cucum-
bers would stay, but not too long. It had two iron doors on it. The food
lasted all winter in there. It was as though you'd just taken them out of
the garden.*

*We had one cow. My mother would get up (you know, the Jewish
men—the Jewish women would always cater to them) and she'd say,
"Shluff, shluff," [sleep, sleep] and go out and milk the cow. I used to
get mad at her: "Why in the world can't Pa do those things?" My
mother did everything: feed the chickens, milk the cow, take care of
the gander, take care of the dogs, everything! I was the oldest of seven
children. So I had to work just like my mother. . . .*

*You know what a mikva is, don't you? A great big [ritual] bath
where the women used to come. They took a great big room and they
turned it into a great big pool. This particular day my mother got
hurt. There was a woman supposed to come for the mikva, and my
mother said, "You better take care of her." Well, I was over 14 years of
age, and I didn't want anything to do with the dirty women. I said I
don't want to do anything with those women! She said "Here is the
Bible; here is what you've got to say." I went to cheder for a long time.
So the woman came, and she said, "Where is your mother?" "My
mother is sick in bed." "Oh," she said, "I've got to go to the mikva."
Well, I said, "I'll take care of you." She said [in Yiddish], "You're just a
child; you don't know the blessings." But I did, and my mother told me
to put a towel over her head and tell her to go down the stairs, and I
told her that and I was going to do the blessings. This particular time
she said it was too cold, and I told her that she would make it warm,*

and I put the towel on her head, and I said, "Go under" and . . . ooooh! [gestures to indicate she fell in]. *That was some experience that I had. It was terrible! My mother's room wasn't far from this part of the* mikva, *and she said her sides were busting out, she was laughing so much.*

I always said to my mother: "You brought me into the world to be the second mother. I'm the second mother, that's what it is." My mother used to go to the store and leave me with the kids to give them their supper and all. Wednesday nights and Saturdays all day.

Before a woman can have intercourse with her husband, she goes for the mikva. *And when you're a bride, they take you for the* mikva. *I was the only one. None of my sisters went to the* mikva. *They refused because of what I told them. My sister Rose, she never cared for Judaism anyway. They eloped. She married a Jewish man though. . . .*

One time our house was hit by lightning. The barn. The horses came out. The hair on the horses was burning. One horse was all right, the other one had to be killed. It was terrible. I think the thunder and lightning in those days was much worse than it is today. Especially being in the woods like that, and all. My uncle was a wholesale junk dealer, and he'd sell carloads of it. My uncle couldn't write; he came from the old country. I'd go with him to the market. They'd put a stone in the bag and I'd see it, and I'd say, "He did it again," and they'd take the stone out, put their foot on the scale. Oh, it was terrible. All the Russian Jews, Polish Jews, they all lived in the same part of the city, and they'd skinflint everyone. They'd just arrived and they'd get a horse and a wagon and they'd yell, "Rags, rags" [rolls her r's]. *They couldn't even say "rags." They'd call us the Yankees.*

[8]

The Limits of Exchange

Human beings are bound together within societies, and their actions work on each other, creating reactions, responses, rebuttals. This truism about human interaction is the stuff of reciprocity and exchange. In interacting with others, we are exchanging with each other, whether through services, goods, talk, gifts, telephone calls, or party invitations. The human way of reciprocity is universal and known among all age groups. When an infant smiles, the parent responds, and a complex pattern of mutuality begins to emerge in their relationship. When a child misbehaves and the parent withholds a gift or affection, the child knows immediately that his action is linked to the reaction in the parent. This quid pro quo characterizes all of human interaction.

Because relationships are not symmetrical and balanced all the time, reciprocity takes on different forms and directly influences who is more powerful, in control, and superior. Mauss theorized in 1925 that not only is gift giving universal, but the giver is superior to the receiver because the receiver is in the giver's debt until the gift is repaid. Lévi-Strauss (1949) extended this concept to the realm of marriage. Because receiving and giving are cyclical and mutually create indebtedness, humans are bound together. This inherent mutuality is aborted when one side always receives and the other always gives, and there is little or no opportunity for the receiver to repay the giver.

Theorists have shown how reciprocity is important among the elderly. Dowd (1975) postulated that elderly persons in the United States were constrained to exchange compliance (in retirement, for example) for benefits related to pensions, old age assistance, and Social Security. Because their control over social and economic resources decreases, compliance becomes the only thing left to exchange for continued security in the social system. Estes (1979) and Hochschild (1973) also noted how the status of the elderly was related directly to their ability or inability to produce economically. Cross-cultural evidence has shown that elderly persons are able to maintain a fairly high status in society when they have something considered valuable by others to exchange, whether it be customs, skills, historical knowledge, economic resources, or inheritances (Vatuk 1980, Gutmann 1976, Cool 1980, Palmore 1975, Amoss and Harrell 1981, Keith 1982a, James, James, and Smith 1984, Amoss 1981, Glascock and Feinman 1981, Foner 1984, among others). When they have little or nothing considered valuable to exchange, dependency increases, and the value of the old person declines.

Amoss (1981) has a provocative explanation for the degraded status of the elderly in modern times that helps explain the liminal status of the nursing-home resident. Instead of linking the status of the elderly with their economic productivity, she thinks that where the elderly are only associated with "nature" as opposed to "culture" (that is, are considered close to death), they are devalued. Where the elderly possess skills considered valuable by others, they are perceived as close to culture rather than to nature; they thereby avoid the association with death and retain prestige.

Already needy and vulnerable, nursing-home residents are subject to another layer of dependency because they are unable to reciprocate with staff members as adults. The basic fact of life in the nursing home is that residents receive care, and staff members dispense care. The inherent inequality of this relationship underlies all else. The lack of resources with which residents can repay staff members reduces their control and increases their dependency. Given this asymmetrical power balance, staff-resident interactions take on particular forms that dramatize inequality, inhibit resident individuality, and dampen spontaneity. Nonetheless, out of this context, residents actively devise strategies to combat their basically passive situation.

Constraints and Contradictions

Initiates in rite-of-passage ceremonies are the recipients of activities, behaviors, and expectations from other members of the so-

[154]

ciety. They are passive in the sense that they are unable to direct the proceedings of the rituals; they fill the ritual roles that have been established by tradition long ago. They are active, however, in the sense that by their individual efforts, they overcome the obstacles and the crises of the passage and are allowed to pass to the next stage. Not so for the nursing-home residents. The passive role that residents of the Franklin Nursing Home must assume creates certain behaviors and conditions, which are elaborated below.

Residents as Recipients

Franklin residents have their basic needs provided for once they are admitted. Payment to their care givers is indirect whether it is paid by the resident or by Medicaid/Medicare because it is made in two stages: the nursing home is paid, and the nursing home pays its employees. Residents are the objects of care-giving services. They have little, if any, resources to repay or otherwise affect those who provide the care. Their behaviors toward staff members have few consequences: they receive care, food, shelter, and medical attention regardless of their actions. Passivity is encouraged. Residents who complain about conditions trespass the moral rule of reciprocity: if they are not paying, they have no right to object; they have no alternatives.

The anthropological literature on aging documents the extensive network and support systems that poor and disabled aged individuals construct for themselves to fulfill their needs and help each other survive. When aged individuals do not receive institutional care, horizontal networks stretch among them and are maintained through reciprocity (Sokolovsky and Cohen 1981). When care proceeds vertically from staff to residents in the nursing home, there is no incentive for horizontal networks to evolve. On the contrary: there is reason for the individual recipients of care to vie among themselves for more.[1] Wax has written: "One who observes the residents of such a home may be surprised at the relative absence of friendships among people of similar status and years, isolated from family and friends. Yet, friendships, as other human relationships, are built upon reciprocity and those who lack possessions, strength and health have relatively little to exchange with each other. What little they have might still be negotiable, except that in a home where the administration is in control of such great benefits in the form of food, shelter,

[155]

social and medical services . . . what can be given or gained from one's neighbor is miniscule" (1962).

An analogous relationship is that between parents and children. Parents dispense food and security to their children, who exhibit rivalrous behavior toward each other as they compete for more affection and goods from the parents. There is some indication that children in abusive families in the United States are resourceful in ensuring that their physical needs are met. They cooperate to a much higher degree with each other than do children in nonabusive families. Perhaps because they recognize at some level that their basic security is in jeopardy, they evolve ways to take care of themselves, becoming grown up and independent thereby. Perhaps there is more resident-to-resident aid in the truly bad nursing homes. In this relatively good nursing home, however, the incentive for supportive networking among residents is reduced.

Reciprocity and Control

When people can reciprocate with each other, they are able to maintain equality and assert control. The following few examples demonstrate instances in which old people in nursing homes have considerable reciprocity, hence control, in their lives. These cases are contrasted with that of the Franklin Nursing Home.

Kayser-Jones (1981) compared a Scottish nursing home with an American nursing home and found that the residents in the Scottish nursing home had more valuable things to exchange than did the Americans. She concluded that because the Scottish residents had goods to exchange, they had some control over their lives. Each resident in the Franklin Nursing Home who is supported by Medicaid keeps only thirty dollars a month to buy such items as candy or birthday cards for friends, relatives, and occasionally staff. Because national health insurance is a right for everyone in Great Britain, the elderly are not singled out for conspicuous consideration as they are in the United States.[2] The Scottish residents made items, which they used to reward staff members whom they liked. Further, it seemed that because the Scottish staff enjoyed higher pay and status than did their American counterparts, there was less theft of residents' belongings than in the United States nursing home.

In one Jewish-sponsored nursing home in the United States, residents are active in raising monies (Kronenberg 1984). They make contributions to the nursing home, and they buy flowers and presents for those among them who may be hospitalized. This same group makes suggestions to the nursing-home administration, which are sometimes implemented. The budget of the residents' council is unused because the fund-raising activities of the group are successful. Another nursing home for Jewish aged in a major United States city does not accept public funds (Wilson 1983). Community members and residents were active in fund raising there. Many residents worked with local companies that had contracted with the nursing home.[3] The ability to reject public monies allows the nursing home some flexibility and power to make policy decisions that are appropriately tailored to the specific conditions of the resident population. A sephardic nursing home in New York City is another interesting contrast (Hendel-Sebestyen 1969, 1979). Residents there had control and decison-making abilities and even ousted a rabbi whom they did not like.[4]

Franklin residents are penalized twice. Their nursing home is quite different from the ones described above. It may be that Franklin residents are frailer and more limited than are the other residents. Hendel-Sebestyen's research was conducted over twenty years ago. It is also possible that somewhat more was expected of the other residents and that they rose to those expectations. In any case, Franklin residents are unable to exchange commodities deemed valuable by others. With little to exchange, dependency on others for aid is increased. Acceptance of their dependent position and their demand for better services make them seem like greedy children who deserve the fate of living their lives in a nursing home. Conversely, when they try to be independent and refuse supports, staff members are sometimes rebuffed and label them "difficult" as a result.

The actions of Franklin residents have few basic consequences. Their past behaviors minimally affect the future, a fact that helps create the timeless atmosphere of the nursing home. Occupational therapy fills time. While some items made during these sessions decorate the institution and are admired and some items are sold in the gift shop at the home, there is no direct connection between the needlework the residents do and the funds these items may generate. The contribution made by the residents seems symbolic at most.

Sarah Zeldin refuses to accept credit for her needlework because she did not design the piece she made; she merely filled in the spaces. She

[157]

maintains that if the staff member who designed the work will put her name on the finished piece, then she will sign her name to it as well. If the staff member does not sign it, then how can Sarah take all the credit? It seems like charity to her.

Many resent being the object of charity, understanding the gratitude and inferiority that is due in return. For this reason, some of the residents attempt to limit the favors that others do for them.

She would like to go downtown and window-shop. But she has put it out of her mind because she would have to ask one of her relatives or one of the staff members to drive her. How could she pay back her debt to the person in that case? If she hears of someone going downtown, maybe then she'll ask to go along.

The residents may view their restricted resources to repay obligations as scarce vestiges of their humanity. When it becomes impossible to repay and one must be the recipient of care and services, one is reduced to nonhuman physical neediness. Dignity is retained in the ability to pay back and thereby exert some control. Goffman's comments on the nature of work in the total institution are relevant here:

> In the ordinary arrangements of living in our society, the authority of the work place stops with the worker's receipt of a money payment; the spending of this in a domestic and recreational setting is the worker's private affair and constitutes a mechanism through which the authority of the work place is kept within strict bounds. . . . Whatever the incentive given for work, then, this incentive will not have the structural significance it has on the outside. . . . Sometimes so little work is required that inmates, often untrained in leisurely pursuits, suffer extremes of boredom. Work that is required may be carried on at a very slow pace and may be geared into a system of minor, often ceremonial, payments. . . . Whether there is too much work or too little, the individual who was work-oriented on the outside tends to become demoralized by the work system of the total institution. . . . There is an incompatibility, then, between total institutions and the basic work-payment structure of our society. (1961:10–11)

Because residents have little power and must receive, they must be grateful. The responsibility that staff members exhibit toward the residents is also reduced by the constraints on reciprocity. When one can repay nice staff members or visitors, one is able to rely on the other person's mutual sense of responsibility. A person who is unable to tap the other's sense of responsibility attempts to induce guilt, and with time guilt is resented. There is little reason for staff members to feel responsible toward the resident because the staff members' obligations are to their bureaucratic duties.

Further, staff retribution can result when residents are too demanding. In subtle and not-so-subtle ways, staff members neglect or delay doing things. They may allow a resident to wet himself; they may not bother to peel the orange so that he can eat it; they may forget to take him for a walk outside. Staff members can perform their duties superficially and impersonally; they can decide what behaviors are in the resident's best interests or not; and they can withhold information from him. The resident's complaints underscore his childish inability to wait. Resentment caused by the care giving exacerbates victimization of, and entitlement by, residents and increases the wedge between givers and receivers. Those residents who are physically or mentally the most restricted in their abilities to care for themselves are the most at the mercy of the nursing assistants and orderlies who attend them.

Control over the care of one's body is thus limited, as is one's control over one's possessions. There is theft and vandalism in the nursing home. Plaques in the hallways engraved with donors' names are often scratched and disfigured. Notices and announcements on the walls are torn off.

The maintenance man and I are taking the elevator. He points out the framed inspection sticker. "That'll be off before long," he comments glumly. "Everything around here gets marred and wrecked. Disgruntled employees maybe. I don't know."

The fact that theft is prevalent increases the residents' knowledge of their insecurity and inability to control their environment. Everything is stealable. Though wheelchairs are labeled with residents' names in large letters, they are stolen and "borrowed" nonetheless. Clothing items are frequently lost in the laundry. Much of the social workers' time is spent answering phone calls from relatives who are angry that their parents' underwear or new clothing that they bought cannot be located. The social workers are resigned to such disappearances and mix-ups. Theft by employees and theft by residents is supplemented by misplacement and honest mistakes. Because it is difficult to distinguish what is stolen from what is lost, the inability to control such disappearances in the impersonal and unaccountable total institution continues.

Conflicts in Kinship Reciprocity

This group of aged Jews endured great sacrifice so that their children could succeed. The reciprocal obligations of children toward their parents remained unspecified and murky. There are tangled emotions about the responsibility that should or should not be directed by children to their aged parents. These intensely difficult problems are created by American and Jewish ideals of maintaining independence along with that of extending or accepting help. There seem to be many factors involved in the quandaries produced.

Fretwell (1982) has suggested that unresolved separation issues between parents and their children from years before often resurface during crises that arise when the parents become very old. Many aged individuals feel that they must maintain themselves independently without burdening the children. Some residents enter the nursing home as an act of independence. Deciding to be admitted is a way of exerting control over one's physical decline. These residents prefer to receive care from an institution rather than from their children. Moreover, if one opts to go into the nursing home rather than live with one's children, a subtle debt may be incurred: the children may feel obligated to visit him, take him to restaurants occasionally, and perhaps do his laundry. Because the elderly resident has made his sacrifice by entering the institution, the adult child must fulfill his obligation to visit. The guilt of families is often profound. Lappin and Grossman write that when aged parents say they do not want to be a burden to their children, they are not necessarily asserting independence: "Upon further investigation, however, the expression very often reveals a feeling of love, approval and acceptance being the reward to children who invite the parents into their lives despite the injunction" (1982:345).

However much children feel the obligation to help and support their parents, the competing cultural expectation that children need not repay their parents is equally strong, if not stronger. The argument made by Bellah et al. regarding individualism in American life is applicable here. Americans justify fewer of their actions in terms of commitment, responsibility, and interdependence on each other than ever before because of the growing belief in individualism. Americans no longer have a language with which to talk about concepts such as obligation, good will, and sacrifice. "No binding obligations and no wider social understanding justify a relationship. It exists only as the expression of the choices of the free selves who make it up. And should it no longer meet their needs, it must end" (1985:107). And again: "The present ideology of American individualism has difficulty, as we have seen, justifying why men and women should be giving to one another at all. . . . Now we are all supposed to be conscious primarily of our assertive selves. To reappropriate a language in which we could all, men and women, see that dependence and independence are deeply related, and that we can be independent persons without denying that we need one another, is a task that has only just begun" (p. 111). Bellah et al. concern themselves primarily with issues of love and marriage and the relationship to one's religion and one's community. They would find much evidence of the similar push-and-pull attitude between commitment and individualism regarding a person's responsibility toward aged family members.

Myerhoff related that the elderly Jews she studied felt it was "natural" for their children to attend to their own needs; nonetheless, a sense of abandonment is hard to avoid in their accounts. Ambivalence about the necessity for reciprocity remains pronounced and is a conflict that permeates their stories. For example: "Basha's daughter calls her once a week and worries about her mother living alone and in a deteriorated neighborhood. 'Don't worry about me, darling. This morning I put the garbage in the oven and the bagels in the trash. But I'm feeling fine.' Basha enjoys teasing her daughter, whose distant concern she finds somewhat embarrassing. 'She says to me, "Mamaleh, you're sweet but you're so *stupid.*" What else could a greenhorn mother expect from a daughter who is a lawyer?' The statement conveys Basha's simultaneous pride and grief in having produced an educated, successful child whose very accomplishments drastically separate her from her mother" (1979:2). Myerhoff states over and again that her informants miss their children but cherish their independence. They are proud that they do not have to rely on their children, be a burden to them, and live with them. Still, they are hurt: "'No, Rebekah,' interrupted Shmuel. 'It's not worth talking about. He is our son and we are proud of him, but that's his own life, and this is ours. It is a fact of life to be hurt by your children. It doesn't matter how good they

[161]

are. That must be accepted, so if you have only your children in life, you will have only pain'" (p. 48). Furthermore, the people at Myerhoff's senior center realized that they had caused their parents a similar kind of pain by cherishing the independence taught them by their parents. This, plus maintaining the belief that family ties are the strongest ones that exist, make the contradiction very difficult: "They realize, they often say, that children must leave their parents, that they left their own families to emigrate when it was necessary, and so they understand the distance between them and their own progeny is inevitable. But the truth is that they counted family ties as the only completely trustworthy relationships, and it was excruciating to them to be so cut off from kinship bonds. Covertly and almost unwillingly, they occasionally reflected on this, asking, 'Is this what our parents felt like when we left them? Did they deserve such treatment? Do we deserve this?'" (pp. 106–7).

Stories about one's obligation to family circulate among staff members at Franklin too, and reflect a similar ambivalence regarding responsibility and independence. For example:

Minnie, a Jewish staff member, is saying that her sister-in-law insisted on taking in her mother when her mother had her leg amputated. The mother had always told her children that when she got too old, she would go to the nursing home. But when she lost her leg, she begged her daughter to take her in. Minnie's brother was against it; the relationship had never been good between them, and according to him, his mother-in-law had been growing more self-centered through the years. Minnie's sister-in-law consulted the rabbi, who advised her not to take her in, but she did anyway. "Well, it was terrible," says Minnie. The old woman died last year, but the couple nearly divorced in the meantime.

Many staff members express anguish about what to do in the case of an ailing parent. Some say that no matter how good a nursing home is supposed to be, they know from experience that abuses and neglect are common. A staff member resolved her problem this way:

When her father was told he had terminal cancer and would only live six months, she knew that if she cared for her father at home family life would suffer terribly. She'd be up at all hours; she would be exhausted; she'd be unavailable to her family. Where did her obligations lie? She was aware of what happens in nursing homes, and she did not want her father to have to be in one. Finally, she decided: she searched out the best nursing home that she could find, knowing full well that it wouldn't be as good as it was supposed to be. And then she made sure that she would go each and every day and supervise what was being done to her father. She wanted them to know that she was watching them carefully. She would make her requests and complaints loud and clear, and she made sure that her father received good care. It was difficult and exhausting. But she was satisfied that when he died she would have done the very best for him that she could, balancing carefully her obligation to her husband and children and her obligation to her needy father.

In those cultures where old people are able and expected to contribute, mutuality within the family continues and seems less problematic. Family members of the residents at Franklin are torn by competing cultural norms about individualism and relatedness, which result in extreme confusion and guilt and cannot be easily reconciled.

Jewish tradition recognizes the difficulty and the competing pressures between one's obligation to oneself and to one's parents. There are numerous biblical and rabbinic references regarding the care and treatment of the aged, including the warning against abandonment of the elderly by the younger generation (Smolar 1986). As Linzer notes, Judaic writings from the Talmud stress the moral obligations that children have to their parents and also acknowledge the conflict when resources are scarce. Even though the rabbis noted the difficulty, they asserted that families should care for their aged parents. It was a familial, not a communal, responsibility. When aged parents are also dependent and sick, an added problem arises: "The illness of aged parents presented the rabbis with a dilemma. They espoused an abiding value for children to act reverentially and kindly to their ill parents, and a value of independence that discourages the child from devoting one's life to parents" (Linzer 1986:45). Each family has to struggle with the particularities of its own situation; easy reconciliation seems unattainable.

Inhibiting Effects of Asymmetrical Reciprocity

Again, when adults are unable to reciprocate with other adults, their status as full-fledged beings is called into question, and their value to others and to the society is markedly decreased as a result. At

Franklin several behaviors—self-protective and insulating mechanisms of making-do—were generated from the nonreciprocity of the residents' status. The following adaptations reveal patterns of behavior; I have noted exceptions to the patterns where I believe they exist.

The Good Resident

To be perceived as good, reasonable, and sane people, residents seem to have two options open to them. They can do good deeds and go out of their way to act like staff members, or they can be good residents by staying to themselves, not complaining, not arguing, not asking for too much.

She wears a staff card that reads "Sunshine Committee" and is always cheerful and energetic. She needs to stay busy, she says, and furthermore, it makes her feel good if she can visit some of the sick residents "on the other side" and cheer them up a little. So every day, if she feels well, she walks over to the new building, and makes her rounds, welcoming new residents and cheering up the sick ones. She considers herself a social worker; "better than some of them," she maintains.

Ida Kanter, considered remarkable by everyone in the nursing home, maintains autonomy in the nursing home in this way.

Residents are helpful to one another in various ways, within the constraints of the nursing home. One resident always accompanied another resident from the sewing room to her room because the confused resident would lose her way by herself. Residents sometimes answer one another's phone calls and leave messages for one another. Though Mrs. Kanter is an active helper, she is limited by rules and expectations in the nursing home. Residents are not allowed to push a neighbor's wheelchair, for example, because the nursing home would be liable in the event of a fall.

"Supporters" in Gubrium's (1975) less restrictive Murray Manor seemed to have more opportunity and leeway to help one another than do residents at Franklin in the 1980s. Preventing accidents by forbidding residents from pushing one another's wheelchairs may have the unfortunate consequence of limiting the helper's self-esteem (and the bond between helped and helper). As nursing homes have

[164]

become more carefully regulated—and more hospital-like than home-like—this trade-off is a sad result.

Another way of coping in the institution is typified by Gerald Wiedenbaum, who minds his own business, does not argue with anyone, and stays out of trouble. He is proud that he is considered a good resident whom everyone likes. Keeping his needs and wants simple, he likes the food and is delighted when his son brings new suits for him to wear. Limiting his social interactions accomplishes two things: he does not become embroiled in the arguments he sees others involved in, and he guards his privacy and his resources by not exposing them to others. The second factor is important for reasons described below.

Monitoring

Related to being a good resident are other responses to limitations on reciprocity: alert residents monitor themselves and each other for signs of mental deterioration. This scrutiny curtails conversation and idle socialization. It is an ingenious and protective mechanism, but it inhibits the development of sturdy relationships. Talk presents the opportunity to make mistakes. Mr. Wiedenbaum, for example, has difficulty expressing himself. Nervous and self-conscious, he frequently forgets what he was about to say. Talking exposes him to the danger that he will not perform well.

Performing well is important to cognitively alert residents. Because they understand that they are in the lucky minority, they seem to monitor one another as well as themselves for signs of incipient slippage. As if to gain some measure of control or predictability over the fortuitousness of events, they scrutinize themselves and one another. Jokes spring from this mechanism of interaction control: Mrs. Zeldin snaps at me brusquely when I misunderstand what she says, with "Can you hear me? Am I talking Portuguese or what?" Aggressively, she points out memory or logic lapses in me as well as in herself during our frequent conversations. One's control, limited as it is in the nursing home, becomes a valued possession. Rather than squander talk, which may betray one, one restricts one's talk, monitors it carefully, metes it out in small doses. Mrs. Zeldin, often more critical than others, expressed her impatience about how others would wander in their talk or reminisce indulgently, and she seemed hypervigilant about not doing the same herself.

Monitoring and adapting to changes that occur in one's friends and neighbors take strength and flexibility. Many residents seem to attempt detachment so as not to be disappointed when a friend dies or becomes ill. Some also try to respect the feelings of their friends whom they witness becoming sicker. Responses to deteriorating health in others takes sensitivity. For example:

Rose seemed to be getting weak, and her friends were quietly noticing the changes. Finally, she was hospitalized, and when she returned, she was placed on the "other side" in the new building. Her friends want to visit her, but she doesn't want them to because she is so much worse. They respect her wishes and stay away. She is a vain woman, and they know she couldn't stand for them to see what she looks like now.

Nurses remark that new residents often try to make friends after they have begun to settle into the nursing-home routine. But if a friend dies or becomes ill, the new resident then learns that it is dangerous to make friends. Keeping interactions to a minimum protects the self against the emotional trauma of these losses. The emotional distance that staff members keep from residents is similarly self-protective. People-work activities, shifting schedules, and frequent changes in nursing assistant-resident assignment prevent continuity. In these ways the nonenduring nature of resident-staff relationships is perpetuated.

Many behaviors in the nursing home are constrained by the pressure of monitoring, as Howsden (1981) has also noted. Slips of the tongue and other possible early manifestations of mental confusion are given important weight. Residents, therefore, take one another both too seriously and not seriously enough. The ability of a resident to project the self that he wants is curtailed.

Though monitoring is a strategy of self-preservation, it limits viable and spontaneous interaction. Residents' social antennae are exquisitely sensitive to incipient deterioration and interaction proceeds superficially, stopping short for self-protection. As such, monitoring may represent the nursing-home resident's basic defense against, and adaptation to, the institutionalized setting.

Talk Stop

Basic talk is curtailed at Franklin. Disputes, arguments, and mistakes occur when people talk. Linguistic mechanisms are used to accomplish control. As though they expected to be considered rambling and boring, several residents pepper their speech with "enders" such as "And that's all, dear," or "What can I say?" These linguistic enders allow the resident to take the initiative to stop the conversation, sparing the speaker embarrassment if his audience is impatient. If I allowed the pause ensuing after an ender to persist and did not follow up on the resident's invitation to end the conversation, he often continued to talk—until the next ender, which he inserted a minute or so later. This mechanism protects the speaker from seeming unaware that the talk is repetitive or overly long. This talk-stop behavior is adaptive because residents are critical of each other and are often quick to note repetitiveness or other similar traits. But these self-monitoring devices muffle free-flowing talk and create a laborious self-consciousness.

Talk is also restricted because there are few experiences about which one can converse. Evolving, interesting experiences are seen to happen to those outside the institution, not inside. The following situation describes a dramatic contrast:

The nursing home organized an overnight trip to a lake resort. The most able residents were permitted to go. They had a good time. The nurse said that the trip was more successful than shorter trips because the residents did more together for a longer period of time. She remarked that after the trip the residents who had traveled together talked about it for a long time. She had never seen the residents talk about anything for that long; nor had she seen any group of residents endure as a group for such an extended period afterward.

During my fieldwork no trips like this one were undertaken. Without events to experience, there is little to share and little about which to converse. However, other kinds of events and experiences are exploited to full effect. Gubrium (1975) describes how residents talked about the content of one another's phone calls and discussed the news of one another's friends and relatives. Franklin residents did this, too, when they could. A visit to my house prompted Sarah Zeldin to com-

[167]

ment later: "I'm still telling them about that fantastic supermarket we went to. And feeding the geese—I'll never forget how that big one went after your Davy. And stirring the tomato sauce while you were on the phone. I can talk about this visit for a long time!"

Reminiscing also seems to be limited at Franklin. Talk about the past is evidence of a wandering mind or is considered irrelevant. Residents are wary about talking about the past because there are so few people present now who were witnesses to the events described (Myerhoff 1979). Without witnesses for support, residents' talk is often considered exaggerated or unimportant. One needs others to corroborate one's account. Myerhoff found that the Jews at the senior center, in contrast, insisted on recapturing the past in order to reconstitute it and preserve it into the present: "More afraid of oblivion than pain or death, they always sought opportunities to become visible. Narrative activity among them was intense and relentless. Age and proximity to death augmented the Jewish predilection for verbal expression. In their stories, as in their cultural dramas, they witnessed themselves, and thus knew who they were, serving as subject and object at once. They narrated themselves perpetually, in the form of keeping notes, journals, writing poems and reflections spontaneously, and also telling their stories to whoever would listen" (1979:33). At Franklin the opposite occurred: participants distrusted events that had already happened. It should also be said that Franklin residents are older, frailer, and sicker, and altogether less capable of these activities. Myerhoff (1979) organized a history class to generate talk and the sharing of experiences. A reminiscence session was organized at Franklin by two volunteers during fieldwork, but it was unclear whether the participants enjoyed the class or not. The volunteers attempted to "get things going" by using artifacts from the past (like an old doll) as stimuli for stories. I heard a complaint that one member of the group always dominated the sessions and that the others seemed alienated. Hazan also relates instances of the elderly rejecting talk of the past: "New participants usually do try to reflect upon their past, but are confronted by an apathetic reaction from the veterans, sometimes accompanied by explanatory remarks such as 'we are here to forget our past not to brood upon it; the Centre is for people who want to forget their troubles' . . . . The realization that the past, even a glamorized one, is irredeemable and irreversible was emphatically reiterated by participants, and they firmly rejected attempts by staff to get them to reflect on it" (1980:90–91).

Idle talk between staff and residents is of low priority, too. Usually too busy to sit down and talk with residents, they have people-work jobs to do. Gubrium's (1975) description of staff members "passing" exchanges in the hallways with residents is reminiscent of many similar exchanges at Franklin: the staff member looks rushed and determined to continue down the hall while he issues formulaic greetings to residents along the way. Though talking is seen as a frivolous activity by most staff members, they sometimes expressed regret that they were unable to get to know the people better. Too often, residents remain unknown, devoid of pasts, identified only with the present physical problems of their bodies.

Active Strategic Responses

Active responses to the lack of reciprocity represent what I consider to be the residents' most positive adaptive strategies.

Bickering

Franklin staff members express distress that many residents dislike and argue with one another. Staff members disagree about the meaning of the hostile behaviors. They assume that the Jewish aged should have much in common and should be friends. Instead they see that residents do not talk with one another or they argue with one another or express jealousy and resentment. Bennett described this phenomenon in the nursing home: "Interaction among residents is generally formal and cordial; great intimacy and intensity of feeling about one another rarely seem to arise. Occasionally, however, there are outbursts of open conflict between residents, particularly between roommates and tablemates" (1962:120). Of course, it should also be remembered that many of the Franklin residents have been unable to get along successfully with others; their presence in the nursing home is a logical outcome of a lifelong failure in relationships. Much of the bickering here seems to revolve around asserting superiority over others or denigrating what are perceived to be others' achievements.

Mrs. Samuels was anxious. The social worker had been talking with her about relaxing. Today Mrs. Samuels gives the social worker a big smile, prompting the social worker to comment that Mrs. Samuels seems much better today and is proud that she seems less anxious. A resident sitting nearby smirks and says, "What a baby you are," about Mrs. Samuels.

Jealousy of others is commonplace.

Sarah Gobin had an invitation to visit a couple of nieces in Florida for a few weeks during the winter. Everyone was overjoyed for her. As she was making excited preparations for the trip, the social worker and administration informed her that because of potentially over-zealous state-inspection procedures that might occur while she was away, she should be prepared to return at one day's notice. If it was discovered that Mrs. Gobin was on a pleasure vacation, her Medicaid eligibility might be in jeopardy. It was just Mrs. Gobin's bad luck that the nursing home was instituting such a policy to safeguard future Medicaid eligibility of its residents. Mrs. Gobin was upset, and one of the things that irked her the most was that another resident had just returned from a glorious vacation in Florida. "Why me?" was all she could ask. "It's not fair that she got to have a vacation and not me."

Myerhoff refers to the sense of injury that her informants had about their basic condition, despite the brave fight they continually waged: "Solipsism is a certain mark of those too long abused. A rainy day is an unkind attack, a broken zipper a manifestation of the hostility of the universe. . . . Such misfortunes, minute in other people's lives, were enormous in theirs. . . . However adept at asserting their independence, disguising their hurts, protecting their pride, they were deeply injured by their situation" (1979:189).

Beyond reflecting injury, bickering indicates for Myerhoff's informants and for many of the Franklin residents better health, and it often signals the germs of community formation. It is rarely found among the sicker residents. It may accomplish several purposes: (1) it keeps people interacting with each other, albeit in negative ways; (2) it keeps people distant from each other; (3) because it protects people from becoming close, it keeps them from losing each other to deteriorating illness and death; (4) it reflects the sense of displeasure that the cognitively aware residents often have about their not-ideal situation; and (5) it may keep people alive. Gutmann (1977) has written that the ability to externalize anger and be aggressive may be linked to the ability to survive. Rather than accept debilitating inner

[170]

conflicts, the individual makes external struggles and finds enemies. Lieberman (1973) has called the same ability "adaptive paranoia" and considers "grouchiness" a survival asset (see also Lieberman and Tobin 1983). The old people turn death into an outer enemy. Staff members at Franklin have discussed this possibility:

At staff conferences there seemed to be some consensus that if one becomes a sweet and loving old person, one's chances of being cared for by an adult child are better than if one becomes an "obnoxious" old person whom no one wants. Nonetheless, in the Franklin population "obnoxious" residents receive more attention than do those who are docile and passive.

Myerhoff (1979) noted that her informants "fight to keep warm." Like the retired people that Keith (1982b) decribed who built community out of their fierce factional political differences with one another, Myerhoff's informants were able to generate crises, prolong disputes, create community discussion on heated issues, and, in so doing, fashion temporary resolutions to the matters that they cared about very much: "Here was a community, then, sewn together by internal conflict, whose members were building and conserving their connections using grievance and dissension. Anger welded them together, fulfilling many purposes at the same time: asserting autonomy over themselves and their circumstances; demonstrating responsiveness to each other; clarifying the community's membership boundaries; displacing resentment from absent, vague targets toward nearer, safer ones; and denying that they shared a common, hideous fate" (1979:187). Disputes and bickering at Franklin, however, seemed to be manifestations of sparks of life that flickered but could not endure long enough to generate community. They remained isolated and small flare-ups of life.[5] Given somewhat better health, slightly sturdier constitutions, and a slightly fiercer determination to persist, these manifestations of anger and unease might have bound these nursing-home residents together.

Strategies to Equalize

Within the confines of the institutional setting, many residents strive to maintain autonomy for themselves and equality with each other and with staff members. The twin goal of autonomy and equality

[171]

is beset with challenges. The resident must be physically and emotionally capable of considerable independence, and he or she must have things or abilities that are valuable to exchange. Kayser-Jones notes how nursing-home residents manage to find ways to assert equality even in their restrictive environments: "Mrs. O'Sullivan has no family, and her closest friend, an 84-year-old woman, lives fifty miles away. Her needs are small; she likes potato chips and mints for snacks and a little wine now and then. Fortunately, she has a skill that she can exchange for service. Mrs. O'Sullivan alters and mends clothes for one of the nurse aides, who in turn shops for her. 'Of course, I wouldn't charge her for it,' she said. 'When I can do her a bit of a favor I do, and when she goes to the store and I need something, she shops for me'" (1981:116).

Some Franklin residents have items that they made or bought that are exchangeable for services. For example, many find it useful to keep candy in their rooms so that they can pay for services that others offer. If one gives candy to the janitor on a regular basis, he may stop at a store on his way to the nursing home to pick up something a resident requests. Because the resident has little to give, however, these exchanges cannot be maintained for long, for the janitor's errands are done primarily on the basis of goodwill. The resulting asymmetry in the exchange usually ensures that it does not endure for long.

Frank, the janitor, has worked at Franklin for many years. He likes most of the residents. Some of them complain all the time, but basically, he sympathizes with them and thinks they are in a tough situation. He used to get things for them whenever certain ones asked. "You get so you know who is going to be asking you all the time." Frank used to pick extra things up from outside on his way to and from work, and they would try to pay him back, but basically they were unable to. He started feeling used. He also found that once he started, the residents wanted more rather than less, so he found himself tangled up doing favors. Finally, he had to tell them no with finality. That's been his policy since.

The "strategy of intimacy" of Myerhoff's (1979) informants allowed Myerhoff to become deeply involved with them. The strategy of intimacy that Franklin residents use often backfires because they have little to exchange with the staff members and because it is a pseudo-intimacy. Guilt often alienates rather than binds.

[172]

Bertha Hyman has been a resident in the wing for three years. She has a nice relationship with one of the recreational therapists. But the recreational therapist has withdrawn from contacts with Mrs. Hyman because she feels an indefinable pressure from Mrs. Hyman to do more than she has already. The recreational therapist doesn't like feeling guilty toward this resident. She finds herself just having less and less to do with her.

Another staff member related the opposite problem:

"Somehow I got involved with Utka Markoff and her brother Abe Alexander. After years of doing this kind of work and warning myself not to become too deeply involved, it happened with these two people. Now I can't extricate myself," she says with a sigh. Somehow, the staff member started doing their laundry, and she still does. She does errands for them, and they call her on the telephone quite often. She feels drained by the situation and doesn't know how to end it.

Occasionally, however, a resident can truly give to a staff person:

Mrs. Safrin related how a nurse from the pool was on duty last night. She didn't know where anything was located on the floor because she hadn't been in the nursing home before. She seemed to be in her mid-forties, Mrs. Safrin thought. From her room Mrs. Safrin overheard several of the residents asking the nurse for this and that, and they were asking impatiently. When the nurse came in to check on Mrs. Safrin, Mrs. Safrin invited her in for a chat. After protesting that she couldn't afford the time to sit and talk, the nurse relented, and after a few minutes of Mrs. Safrin's soothing approach, the nurse began to confide the troubles of the day. Mrs. Safrin was sympathetic and offered the nurse a plant to take home with her. "No one ever gave me a plant before," exclaimed the nurse to Mrs. Safrin's disbelieving ears. Mrs. Safrin related the story with much pride.

How often residents lend a comforting ear to beleaguered staff members is unclear. Staff members may view some residents as able confidants who are understanding and "safe."

Relationships between residents and staff members are subsumed under the unequal staff-resident barrier of the nursing home which prevents an enduring friendship, however. Duties of the job, profes-

[173]

sional demeanors of all sorts, and the numerous federal and state rules determine to a large degree the behaviors between staff and residents.

Mrs. Zeldin feels fortunate that the nurse who is usually on duty at night will allow her to take the aspirin she requires for her headaches at her own discretion. But she realizes that the nurse is letting her determine her own timing out of goodwill, which she could retract at any time. In fact, Mrs. Zeldin knows that she also places the nurse in some jeopardy by appealing to her goodwill in this matter. She feels at the mercy of these rules and the likely changes in nurse behavior that may ensue.

Mrs. Zeldin is in the kind of situation that might prompt her to give gifts to the nurse so that the nurse is indebted to her. Then Mrs. Zeldin would have some assurance that the nurse's willingness to let her take aspirin at her discretion would continue.

Attempts by residents to blur the boundary between residents and staff can be thwarted. Therefore, residents who try to equalize the relationship risk failure and possible damage to their self-esteem. When a resident attempts to equalize the relationship, the staff member may refuse. The result is that both parties have dramatized the inherent inequality between them. The split is thus more apparent after such an attempt, as when Max Sager attempted to offer a glass of wine to the social worker, thinking they enjoyed a symmetrical friendship, and she refused.

Even though the risk of failure accompanies resident attempts to equalize relations with staff members, the risk may be worth taking for the successes that sometimes result. Furthermore, as has been shown, it may benefit some staff members to blur the distinction between the residents and themselves for the comfort and reassurance they can sometimes receive.

Getting Needs Met

Residents must tread a fine line. In order to obtain the things they desire and need, they must be persistent but not too demanding. Most residents know that they will be ignored if they do not issue reminders, but their efforts will be denied, thwarted, or delayed if they persist too impatiently. For some, being ignored is its own reward. Maintaining a cheerful exterior and remaining in reasonable health ensures one a certain anonymity behind which one can do things according to one's wishes.

A resident puts newspapers on the open windows on these hot summer days to have shade as well as ventilation. The administrator has told her not to do it because it does not look good from the street, but she does it anyway because the heat is unbearable in these non-air-conditioned rooms. When he protests, she takes them down, and then puts them up another time. They each go through their motions, she says.

Goffman refers to this kind of strategy in total institutions as "make-do's" (1961:208).

"Forgetting" a rule that seems trivial and continuing to do something one's usual way is an example of using a deficit to maximum efficiency, provided it is managed skillfully. Strategies such as not remembering and not hearing can, when selectively used, be instrumental in making sure that certain needs are fulfilled according to one's wishes. Acting as if one needs help can often provoke the aid desired. There is a fine line, then, which staff members often find hard to distinguish, between a resident's actual ability to do something and his inability to do it.

The staff discussion about Jacob Strauss is almost over. One of the staff members asks why Mr. Strauss is in a wheelchair. No one seems to know. He has been here so long, no one can date when he started using a wheelchair and why he uses it. "Can he walk or not?" asks the medical director. No one knows for sure.

In another resident-care conference it is learned that a female resident has most of her grooming tasks taken care of by her nursing assistants.

"Can't she brush her hair by herself?" someone asks the nursing assistant. The nursing assistant is not sure. There is disagreement among the staff about whether the resident should be encouraged to brush her own hair or whether it is important to brush the woman's hair as an expression of closeness. Though it is decided that the woman should be urged to brush her own hair, some of the staff members still feel that giving in to the woman's wishes to have her hair brushed by them should be allowed.

This incident raises a difficult and persistent quandary in the nursing home: how to provide aid and support in a humane way without promoting dependency. Indulging the resident too much is one extreme; expecting no dependency is the other. It is to this nursing home's credit that the issue is debatable and considered problematic in the resident-care conference.

Sometimes a resident strategy is tolerated (and misunderstood) as a harmless and strange quirk that old people have.

Bernice Meyerhov takes sheets from the closet near her room. She does it when she thinks no one is noticing. The nurses know she takes them, and they do not stop her. She needs to have the extra sheets on hand in order to change her incontinent brother's bed in the night. The nurses think Mrs. Meyerhov has a strange hoarding behavior.

There are dozens of reasons every day that residents cannot be treated the same. They have different needs, and changes occur constantly. Rules that ensure a uniform policy for everyone always founder on the fact that needs are idiosyncratic, and individuals have varying skills in obtaining what they want.

Ralph, the maintenance man, says this is the rule: If you have a light bulb out, or if a shelf needs to be propped up, or if you need your television stand raised, or if something needs to be fixed in the bathroom, you submit a work order to Tom Mills, the head of maintenance. Tom assigns his men according to the order that the jobs come in. That's only fair. But the residents are always messing up the system. When Ralph goes down the hall with a light bulb for Mrs. Kahn's room, for example, Mr. Bell requests that Ralph replace the bulb in his room too. Mrs. Kahn put in the work order properly, and Mr. Bell only thought of it now. This kind of thing gets Tom really mad.

It is an inefficient system, and it makes sense to the residents that Ralph fix two light bulbs at the same time, rather than one today and one next week. It makes sense to Ralph, too, and he is frustrated to be caught in the middle.

Asking nicely and having a sense of humor aids one's ability to get what one wants:

[176]

Mrs. Safrin told Tom that when she sat on her throne, she felt a strong breeze from the window. This was her nice way of informing Tom that she wanted her bathroom window fixed since on these chilly fall days she was cold when she used the toilet.

Mrs. Safrin did not want to use up the limited amount of goodwill that she knew she carried with these men. She asked them to adjust a shelf in her room. They did it, but then when she opened her trunk, the lid did not go all the way up. She asked them to adjust it again, and they did, but then something else did not work after that. She decided not to request anything else for a while and to make do with the way it was.

Residents make their wishes known according to hierarchies present in the total institution. There are channels that they are supposed to use and that they often subvert.

Mr. Strauss has been in the nursing home for years. He has no patience for the hierarchical system, which works too slowly for his purposes. When he wants something, he asks the nursing supervisor directly. Because she happens to like him, she does what he asks. However, the charge nurse on Mr. Strauss's floor is angry that he goes over her head to the top of the hierarchy. The nurses feel that the nursing supervisor should redirect Mr. Strauss to the proper channels, but she never does. Mr. Strauss obtains what he wants.

Similar difficulties attend residents' desires to change dietary or medical restrictions of various kinds.

A resident appealed directly to the administrator about his food complaints rather than go to dietary, thus embarrassing the dietician.

Such tactics can be detrimental to the resident because they serve to alienate the staff. Sometimes, however, they are effective: a resident must go outside the established hierarchies carefully in order to obtain what he wants without angering key people.

The ability to have needs and desires satisfied is enhanced when a resident has resources on the outside. Family members who are actively involved with the resident and his care represent an advantage to the resident. Thus, as was described in an earlier chapter, not only does having a family member do one's laundry, go on errands, and appeal to staff members on specific matters directly aid the resident, but the supportive resources also make clear the higher status of the resident.

Touching

Touching is probably the main mechanism for positive interaction in the nursing home. It is pervasive; it is explicitly taught to staff members; it is often spontaneously practiced. When the social worker talks to a resident, she holds the resident's hand tightly, often touching the resident's back or shoulders or hair with her other hand. In physical therapy the sense of touch is one of crucial support. Therapists lift and carry, support, grab, press, and urge the residents in various physical ways to try harder for results. Behavior at Franklin corroborates Weinberg's (1976) assertion that as "visual and auditory acuity diminish and the environmental language becomes less discernible," the elderly have an increased need for intimacy and touch. The strength in the hands of many of these old people is impressive. Time after time I was held in viselike grips during greetings or conversations.

More physical contact of this kind would seem beneficial. For example, the medical director's physical contact with the individual resident he interviews is quite pronounced. He leans dramatically forward so that his face and the resident's face are extremely close. He clasps both of the resident's hands in his. Sometimes he holds one hand and puts his other arm around the resident's shoulder in an embracelike, enclosing gesture. Other staff members are often astonished at the responsiveness of the resident in these interviews. "I've never known him to be so 'with-it,'" exclaimed one nurse after an interview with a usually taciturn and confused resident, indicating the effectiveness of this physical approach and the heightened performance aspect of the interview setting.

Residents touch each other frequently. They shake hands and touch while they talk. To compensate for hearing loss, residents lean toward each other closely, and touching seems a natural accompaniment. For those residents whose physical deterioration is great, touching is the last and most primary link. One social worker who had an important relationship with a female resident described her feelings:

[178]

"Mrs. Glasgow was a very vain woman. She always wanted to be dressed prettily and have her hair look nice. As she became more ill, she withdrew from people more. I felt that she didn't want them to see how she had become. She let me sit with her, hold her hand, brush her hair, and tell her how lovely she looked. She knew she was going to die. She told me. I felt the only important thing I could do was be with her and brush her hair. I knew that was meaningful to her."

The social worker expressed satisfaction that she had followed her instincts in this manner, and wished that more staff members followed her practice.

Structurally prohibited from mutuality by being old, frail, and institutionalized, the residents still summon their remaining resources to exert some choice and control where they can. They stay to themselves, watch each other carefully, bicker, complain, and touch, and they eke out ways of getting some satisfaction out of their institutional lives. In a setting where choice and control are thus limited, dependency is basic. It is complemented and deepened by the timeless liminality of the nursing-home experience—a liminality whose time-limitedness remains unacknowledged.

Voice: Bernice Meyerhov

Well, I was born in Russia, Norodich. Norodich, I born there. This is not so big town. And I was raised by my mother and my brothers. I am the oldest. But I was the only girl. And I was raised up in the town. And my town was a small town, and there's not so much work, you know, so you have so many children you need so much, you know. We used to send them to the Jewish school to teach you Jewish. Everybody was very religious—we used to have the teacher in mine own house so we don't pay. He was living in my home. And so you grow up, you grow up, you know. The cheder, *you know. All my brothers were very religious. They used to go to the synagogue. The teacher used to write home, "very nice boy, very nice boy." All my brothers, they help, they were hard workers. My father was far away. I went through a lot. I went through a lot. He couldn't send money.*

My mother. My mother used to make some white bread, and Sunday we used to go to the church and the Russians used to come in, the goyim *used to come in, and we would give them the bread and some schnapps. We were supposed to have a license. We used to get a little fish. My mother used to have a little store, and the Russian people used to catch some fish, bring the fish, and we'd weigh it on the scales, so many pounds. This was wholesale, my mother used to buy wholesale. Then my mother would sell it to make a profit. So that's how we'd do it during the war. One brother used to make the leather—what do you call it?—he used to make the holes, make the leather outside. Two brothers used to make the patterns from the leather. And then people used to come and they would pay him. They were quite young. They were not married yet, still single. This was when my father was away.*

They would help out because everything in Europe was very high. We used to have a cow. We used to buy food for the cow. We had to buy wood. So my mother had to go every time to the Russian people—they would bring wood in the packet. Oy! Oy! So much. We used to buy the wood and keep it outside. The Russian people used to go around and my mother used to hire them to chop the wood. We used to have a special room to put the wood. And when it's cold we would burn it. What can I say? There are so many things I remember, but. . . .

My home had five rooms. For my brothers, for me and my mother one room, and then one room for the teacher. And the kitchen. Our water was outside. My husband—me and my husband—we grow up together—we hired a man to make a well. And we hired a woman and she used to bring us water. Every Monday we used to have a bath— me and my mother—a special bath. The men they used to go on Friday because Friday was Shabbos. Me and my mother, we used to go with other women. It was in another place, not our home—near the river. Used to be a big lake. So we used to go there. We used to bring hot water and we used to wash. Oy! I didn't remember to tell you how much I went through. What can I say?

On Shabbos my father used to come home early. At 12:00 we used to prepare. Some meat—we used to have soup mit lochshen—noodles— meat—and we used to have dessert—apples. "Good Shabbos," every-one used to say. *My mother used to go to the synagogue, everyone used to go to the synagogue. . . . "Good Shabbos."*

Everybody they kill. The goyim. The Russians. So anyway, Oy! On Shabbos we went to the synagogue. I would hear: "Close the doors. Close the doors—you shouldn't go out. The Russians—the goyim." No Jews would go out. *Inside, we were hiding because outside—the Russians were outside. I was a young girl. No, I was married. Oy! Don't ask. I had my son, a little boy, and I had a baby. My mother's sister lived in another town, and they came to our town because they were afraid. The only sister that my mother had. She was in bed with a baby. So anyway, so much story. We were worried about my auntie— she was in bed all alone with the baby. And we don't know what happened. I don't know where my brothers are—I don't know where anybody is. Can't remember. The only thing—I was sitting outside with my baby to my breast, and we hear the Cossacks. On the other side they started to kill—so many—and we hear "Gevald! Gevald!"* [help!] *we hear. So anyway I took my baby and we used to go to a Russian who was good to us. Oy! I ran away. This time was summer. I*

[181]

was married. I used to run with my baby to a Russian, a friend of my mother's—to hide us—because he's a goy. Maybe he could save us. So I came in and I beg him, "Let me in!" And he said no because when they come they'll see that he is hiding. So he said, "In the garden, in the garden." And it was summertime. He said, "Hide in the sweet corn"—afraid maybe they're going to kill him because he hide Jews— yidden. So I took my baby and I took my boy and I hide in the sweet corn. And it was near to my house and I hear how they kill people. You hear, "Gevald!" After a while it was quiet and the man said, "I think they went away now." So I came out with my children and I find my mother. We were crying. I don't know where my brothers. I don't know where my husband. Are they alive? Oh! What can I say? They ran away—they were afraid—they expect to be killed. What can I say? So much to talk—I can remember so much. The goyim came back the same day. They took their money. Ach! My brothers and my husband say that with our money—from the leather—from the skin of the cows—maybe if we give them money they don't kill us. Oy! So they came in and I say I have no money. They didn't kill. It's not enough how much I tell you. There's still so much to tell you. How we took up all our things and we went away from Norodich. My father said, "You should come."

[9]

Liminality in the Nursing Home: The Endless Transition

Consider marriage, a typical rite of passage: engagement marks the couple's momentous decision to change their private relationship into one that is public and official. No longer is each person considered single. The ring, excited announcements, newspaper notices, gifts, parties, and preparations for the wedding are symbols and activities that mark the engagement. The couple is nervous. Jokes and stories from others make the couple into willing victims and teach the couple about what awaits them in marriage. The couple is reminded that it is not too late to back out. Bachelor parties tease the couple about the single life it has left. The wedding ceremony formally and publicly incorporates the couple as married. It ends the threshold, in-between state of the engagement.

Engagement in this example is the liminal portion of the rite of passage. Separated from his old role and not yet installed in his new role, each person is suspended. Dependency, excitement, anxiety, and cameraderie are heightened. Turner has written:

The subject of passage ritual is, in the liminal period, structurally, if not physically, "invisible". . . . the symbolism attached to and surrounding the liminal *persona* is complex and bizarre. . . . They are at once no longer classified and not yet classified. . . . The metaphor of dissolution is often applied to neophytes. . . . The other aspect, that they are not yet classified, is often expressed in symbols modeled on processes of gestation and parturition. The neophytes are likened to or treated as embryos, newborn infants, or sucklings by symbolic means which vary from culture to culture. . . . The essential feature of these symbolizations is that the neophytes are neither living nor dead from one aspect, and both

[183]

living and dead from another. Their condition is one of ambiguity and paradox, a confusion of all the customary categories. (1967:95–97)

On communitas, the positive feeling of togetherness that initiates share with one another, Turner has explained:

> If complete obedience characterizes the relationship of neophyte to elder, complete equality usually characterizes the relationship of neophyte to neophyte, where the rites are collective. . . . The liminal group is a community or comity of comrades and not a structure of hierarchically arrayed positions. This comradeship transcends distinctions of rank, age, kinship position, and, in some kinds of cultic group, even of sex. . . . Deep friendships between novices are encouraged. . . . All are supposed to be linked by special ties which persist after the rites are over, even into old age. . . . This comradeship, with its familiarity, ease and, I would add, mutual outspokeness, is once more the product of interstructural liminality, with its scarcity of jurally sanctioned relationships and its emphasis on axiomatic values expressive of the common weal. . . . The passivity of neophytes to their instructors, their malleability, which is increased by submission to ordeal, their reduction to a uniform condition, are signs of the process whereby they are ground down to be fashioned anew and endowed with additional powers to cope with their new station in life. (1967:100–101)

The liminality of nursing-home life—between adult life in the community and death to come—is different. Like other liminal states there is dependency and separation, but unlike other liminal states the dependency is not accompanied by teaching, preparation for the next stage is actively discouraged, religion and ritual are minimal, involvement by the community is meager, and isolation is prevalent. There is little cameraderie or ceremonial notice to accompany this transition. Nursing-home residents begin their last rite of passage aided neither by already socialized nursing-home residents, by staff members of the nursing home, nor by individuals from Harrison. Thus this rite of passage accentuates the lonely aspects of liminality, and resolution is secured only by the physical fact of death.

Separation

Entering the nursing home is accomplished by a series of leave-takings or separations. Separation creates the liminality of the transi-

[184]

tion, the neither-here-nor-there state that makes the initiate receptive to teachings about the next stage. In the nursing home, however, the separation is accomplished for its own sake. Instead of tasks and preparation work for reincorporation into a new status, there are security and assurances about the transition itself. The Jewish community, the medical community, and the nursing community exhibit ambivalent attitudes toward the nursing home and its residents. The services provided in the nursing home decrease the need for the residents to secure those same services in the community. Dependency on the institution is ensured, and one is cut off and made passive.

Total institutions need not necessarily be separate from the community in which they are located. As was indicated earlier, some residents from one nursing home work in local businesses. A Jewish orphanage operated during the first half of this century in a city approximately the same size as Harrison provides an interesting comparison (Michel 1977). Its administrators included the children in as many community activities as possible. They attended religious school at the nearby temple, and they went to the local public schools. They were encouraged to visit the homes of children from the schools and to stay overnight whenever invited. The children participated in activities such as the Boy Scouts and the local summer camps. There were trips downtown to visit Santa Claus at Christmastime. Overall, a conscious effort was made to deinstitutionalize the orphanage and to allow the children to be as "normal" as other children. Integration of the Franklin Nursing Home into the community today does not seem to be valued.[1] While it seemed necessary for the children to learn the social skills that would enable them to enter the community as they grew older, today, elderly individuals are not expected to maintain continuity with their lifetime roles, memberships, and contacts. The separation is assumed: one leaves behind a past life. For all symbolic and practical purposes, the continuity is severed.

Time

Time is often described as endless or strange in liminal states. In the nursing home a sense of timelessness coupled with various rigid staff routines creates a unique institutional time. Time looms large. It seems unfillable and is fraught with peril. It needs to be broken up because days and weeks seem the same. Certain strategies allow residents to get through the days and the weeks, much as "passing time" occupied the residents of Murray Manor (Gubrium 1975). While the more intact residents manage their time more individually than do the less capable residents, continual exposure to the deterioration of others and the steady knowledge of one's own closeness to death lend a particular edge to the perception of time in the nursing home.

Time Routines for More Capable Residents

Time is tracked by the secular calendar, by the Jewish calendar, by clock, and by nursing shifts. Knowledge of what day it is is necessary to predict visits, telephone calls, outside doctor visits, and events relevant to family members. Residents also know staff time because it affects their lives directly. Much time is spent sleeping and watching television.

I was looking for Max Isaacs, the resident who had been admitted only two weeks earlier. When I knocked on his door, he called, "Come in," and as I went in his room, he was rising from his bed. I saw that I had disturbed his nap. He explained that it was all right; he naps on and off throughout the day. Numerous other times when I was looking for him after that, I found him either napping in his room or napping in the lounge downstairs.

Meals, activities, visits, telephone calls, and other events further structure the day. One well resident, Ella Stein, describes her day as follows:

"Usually I wake up when Esther [the LPN] gets here early in order to find a parking space, and she lies in bed next to me for about fifteen minutes before the shift begins. So that's a little before 7:00. Sometimes I've slept pretty well during the night, but more often I've been sleeping off and on, thinking about things, remembering, you know. After I get up and get dressed, water my plants, and spend time in the bathroom, sometimes I turn on the TV or do my rounds. I don't spend much time, I just check up on people, see how they're doing. Then I come back here, and I always keep the door a little bit open so I can see what's happening on Fifth Avenue. Then we're waiting for the [food] truck. It's usually about 9:30. There's no use in going to the dining room before I hear the truck because then I just have to sit

around and wait. Just more chance to get in a fight with someone. A few minutes after the truck goes by, that's when I go down.

After breakfast she goes to the front lobby to see what is doing there; usually she buys a newspaper and checks the obituary page. She goes early to physical therapy to avoid seeing the sick residents who arrive later. Then she goes to the needlework session and spends a few hours there. Soon it is time to go back to her room; she usually watches a soap opera until she hears the truck go by. After lunch she watches more soap operas.

Sarah Zeldin refers to her contacts on the outside by the days that she may typically see them. Thus, she has a "Saturday cousin" and an "every-other-Wednesday-lunch niece" and a "Tuesday-morning-volunteer visitor." She is grateful for these visits and recognizes with icy exactness how dependent she is on their continued goodwill in making these visits to her. She also understands that the nature of these visits and contacts is that they decrease with time: "My Wednesday-lunch niece used to come every week. After a while, these lunches became every-other-Wednesday lunches. Every now and then, she calls and cancels. I can't blame her; she has her own life, and she can't ignore her family. It's been quite a few weeks since I've seen her. She might be calling tomorrow."

Other well residents structure their days according to their own routines. The meals are the important signposts during the day. Each person has his own way: a time to read the newspaper, watch television, sit in the lobby, visit others, take a walk, attend favorite activities, go to physical therapy, take a nap.

Stanley Fierstein stays busy, and he has disdain for those who "waste" their time by sleeping and sitting. He takes vigorous walks, dresses carefully, attends certain activities, and visits his children for meals or overnights. Ida Kanter structures her day according to her various tasks: Depending on how strong she feels, she has a certain way of making her rounds throughout the wing and the new building. There is a lot of territory to cover to visit new or sick residents.

Charlie Kassin has his rounds as well.

Up early, he walks throughout the nursing home, covering most or all of the floors before his breakfast. Right now he is checking on his cousin, Freida Kleinberg. He has heard from some of the nurses that she is eating very reluctantly, and he is giving her his daily morning pep talk to have a good breakfast.

Time Routines for Less Capable Residents

Sicker residents have less control over the structure of their days. They are, to varying degrees, the passive recipients of routines performed on them by different staff members. Many of the residents become anxious as they anticipate the change in shift.

The charge nurse on the third floor is describing how the atmosphere of the floor changes at about 2:30 in the afternoon. Many of the nursing assistants, orderlies, and nurses are lolling around the nurses' station, some are already in their coats, and they're chatting with one another animatedly, appearing restless to go home. At the same time, the new shift is coming on, and there are greetings and personal catchings-up that go on between members of the two shifts. Various residents are acting more disturbed at this time; they appear restless; they repeat their questions with urgent frequency; they are less soothed by reassurances.

Knowing who is "on," whether someone has the day off, or whether the day will somehow be structured differently is important, especially to those residents who rely exclusively on their nursing assistants and orderlies for the minute details of their lives. They are informed that today there will be a visit to the doctor. Later, they are wheeled to lunch, and after lunch, perhaps, transported to the first floor for bingo or a party. At different times during the day, depending on their condition, they may be taken to the bathroom, or put to bed, or transferred from bed to chair, or bathed. Resident attempts to alter staff schedules in their care meet with little success. A resident's frequent requests to talk to the nurse, or have his shower early, for example, are brushed off as annoying interruptions.

Mr. Allen came down the hall again, still in his bathrobe. "May I speak to a nurse, please?" he asked. No answer from the four personnel at the nurses' station. Two of them are charting; two others are in conversation with each other. After a few more tries, one of the nurses looks up and asks Mr. Allen what he wants. "May I please have my shower now?" he asks. The nurse explains, with some irritation, that Ned, his orderly, is on his break now, and he will have his shower later on in the afternoon.

Resident time management usually succumbs to staff schedule and staff whim rather than to resident needs.[2] A resident's wish to be taken out of bed later in the morning may be refused because if he is not made ready for breakfast at a certain time, the nursing assistant will not be able to get the other residents in her charge ready in time. Therefore some residents will be awakened an hour or more before breakfast, and they will have to sit, sometimes in great discomfort, in a chair before breakfast is served. Gubrium describes the routine at Murray Manor in this way:

> Aides take patients to the dining room three times a day. Breakfast necessitates the most extensive bed-and-body work, since many patients must be awakened and dressed before the meal. Some premeal events slow down bed-and-body work. For example, patients may insist on being taken to toilet or having the bedpan when an aide is ready to take them to the dining room for lunch or supper. Or someone may soil his clothing in such a way that it is difficult to hide from anyone or pass off as unnoticed. Once patients are in the dining room, food is not served immediately. Typically, those patients who have been taken there first because "they're not complainers" sit in their wheelchairs or regular chairs at the table for some time. They wait through two premeal events before they eat. First, they wait through the time it takes the floor staff to get all patients who are scheduled to eat in the dining room seated there. This ranges anywhere from a half-hour to a full hour. Second, they wait for their food trays to arrive from the kitchen. (1975:129–30)

Laird describes her dilemma during her own nursing-home stay: "Now I was torn by one of those deep concerns over trivia which typically afflict persons dependent upon the services of others. I wanted to be got up 'sooner' because I frequently had urgent need to use the toilet; and 'later' because the longer I could stay in bed, the shorter would be my often agonizing 'sit' in the wheelchair" (1979:64). Similar constraints attend bathroom routines. Those residents who are not incontinent but who have difficulty walking must rely upon their nursing assistants and orderlies to bring them to the bathroom.

Freida Kleinberg expresses her horror of becoming more dependent because she will be at the mercy of the timing of whatever staff mem-

[189]

ber is on duty. Imagine having to wear a diaper or wait to be taken to the bathroom!

Ideally, nursing assistants and orderlies are supposed to take the residents in their care to the bathroom every two hours. Whether the residents are taken to the bathroom often depends on how many residents the staff person is assigned to that day. The particular timing of the bathroom visit is only sometimes determined by the resident.

"Will you take me to the bathroom, please?" asks Mrs. Behrenbaum. After she repeats this request quite loudly, a nursing assistant calls over to her, "I'm not your aide. Wait till Bertha comes back."

The sick residents' access to activities and special events held during the day is restricted by the availability of staff personnel both to transport them to the activities and to keep the floor adequately covered. The particulars of lunch schedules, break times, and how many staff personnel are on duty in any particular day determine whether an individual may or may not go to an activity, especially if the resident himself is unable to remember that an event is taking place.

Contact with family also structures time. Regular evening visits with a son or a daughter can be anchoring for the resident, both emotionally reassuring and temporally orienting. Receiving or placing daily telephone calls is another way of marking time and filling it.

"Is it time to call my daughter now?" Mrs. Deutsch asks Sarah Zeldin, anxiously. "No, dear," answers Mrs. Zeldin, patiently. "You always call her after lunch. We haven't had lunch yet. I'll remind you. Don't worry."

Staff time accounts for the large differences between day, evening, and night shifts and between weekday and weekend. Few staff members are on duty during the evenings, nights, and weekends. Because social workers and activity personnel are not present to structure the time into events, the time seems unbroken and long. Staff members are less supervised; there is more neglect of residents. Residents with interested family members visit with them at these times, either inside the institution or outside. Residents who are not visited by family or friends are doubly isolated at these times.

[190]

Time of Future Peril

Exposure to deterioration and death is a continual accompaniment to life in the nursing home. Residents seem to be matter of fact about it. Cognitively intact residents bluntly acknowledge their closeness to increasing disability and death. They say things such as: "Well, we're all here to die." "Obviously, this is the last stop." "I hope I'll have a chance to pick some of your grapes, if I'm around in the fall, that is."

Hochschild notes how the old have become society's "shock absorber" of death: "Because in America one age group is divided from another, confining friendships within age boundaries, it is the old whose friends die. If friendships outside the family were evenly distributed throughout the age scale, young people would face loss through death as much as old people do. As it is, the old have become a 'buffer zone' between society and death" (1973:86). Like the widows of Merrill Court that Hochschild describes, the residents of Franklin are not buffered from death. Many residents see their fate clearly in the other residents around them. Residents who live on the self-care unit witness their neighbors become sick, go to the hospital, and either die there, come back well enough to retake possession of their old room, or come back at a lower level of functioning, necessitating that they thereafter live in the new building "on the other side." It is a reality that most of the residents acknowledge readily. One resident said: "At least I can still walk and talk. But if I have another heart attack, I might end up like him." Another said: "Well, it's fine now. I can take care of myself and not bother anyone and pretty much not be dependent on anyone. But I have to expect that any time, I could end up like Rose, who knows, and go to the other side. That's what I dread. Now I can take my pills by myself if I've got a stomach ache. But what if I were worse, and I had to ask for my pills, and then they took their time in giving them to me. Oh, I pray that it just happens when it's going to happen, in my sleep. We all hope that, you know."

Another sense of time has to do with the timing of death. Some Franklin residents "know" when they are going to die.

A social worker was telling me how active and involved Hy Spielman always had been in the nursing home. But then one day he looked bad, and he told her that he was going to die within the next few days. She tried to joke him out of it, but he was telling her in a straightforward

[191]

and detached way as if he had heard the weather report, and she was impressed with his certainty. He died as predicted.

Incidents such as this one are not considered rare.

The Jewish daycare center in London that Hazan (1980, 1984) studied contrasts with the Franklin Nursing Home. Hazan considers the elderly in "limbo" because of the paradoxical juxtaposition of two conflicting conceptions of time: a static time derived from the welfare system, which gives benefits without repayment, and a deteriorating time caused by the ailments experienced by the aged. Hazan shows how these elderly construct an "alternate reality" of time in which they care for each other and are shielded from the outside. Time in Franklin, on the other hand, betrays the certainty of how limited the time actually is for the residents. The time of "future peril" that intact residents perceive as their fate threatens the quality of resident relationships rather than intensifies them. While the nursing-home staff attempts to protect and shield the residents from the unpleasantness of the reality of death, the residents witness, attempt to distance themselves from, and, ultimately identify with, the inevitability of death.

There are several different kinds of time, then, at Franklin. There is the cyclical time of the day and of the week, which is marked by regular changes of the nursing shift and punctuated by planned activities. Concurrently, there is static time in which everything seems the same. One day appears like the rest; the time is empty, and the task is to fill it. There are the calendar references to secular and Jewish events, which structure time and provide one of the few means to create an anticipation of the future. And there is the time perception of future peril: that with each passing day, the risk of experiencing more deficits and of requiring increased care is greater and is witnessed continually in others. However, this time of future peril is fought by staff denial and cylical institutional routines. This contradiction intensifies rather than resolves the ambiguity of the liminality.

Dependency

Dependency is another marker of liminality. Subjects in rites of passage are often acted upon by other members of the society. The engaged couple, for example, receives gifts and advice, and must wait.

Enduring the transition promotes dependency. In the nursing home, residents guard the independence and evidence of autonomy that they still have, knowing it is a time-limited, precious commodity.

Manifestations of dependency in this country are viewed with shame and are considered portents of worsening dependent behaviors to come. The dependency-down of old age is thus different from the dependency-up of childhood. As Clark wrote about the cultural meanings of dependency: The possibility of dependency in old age is a frightening prospect to most Americans. It has been remarked that our definition of freedom is based on a sweeping faith and confidence of the individual in his own competence and mastery. Only by being independent can an American be truly a person, self-respecting, worthy of concern and the esteem of others. In applying this notion to the case of the aged, it seems that this particular cultural imperative, in the end, forces many elderly people in our society to make an unhappy choice between denial of need for help, on the one hand, and self-recrimination on the other" (1973:82). A dependent adult is viewed as sick, weak, nonadult, or all of these. Because he is sick, the dependent old person is exonerated for his lack of responsibility but he is also excluded from his former stature as an adult.[3]

In excruciating detail, anthropologist Robert Murphy describes the countless logistic struggles in his daily life and how he has had to deal with, and acknowledge the identity of, the dependency into which quadriplegia has forced him: "Lack of autonomy and unreciprocated dependence on others bring debasement of status in American culture—and in many other cultures. Most societies socialize children to share and reciprocate, and also to become autonomous to some degree. Overdependency and nonreciprocity are considered childish traits, and adults who have them—even if it's not their fault—suffer a reduction in status. This is one reason why the severely disabled and the very old often are treated as children. . . . It is for these reasons that escape from dependency has been a central goal of the disability political movement, and many handicapped people have discovered their own possibilities through going it on their own" (1987:201).

Initiates in rites of passage are made dependent by the event, but this dependency seems to have the purpose of preparing the initiates for the next stage. There are teachings and tasks, and learning may be facilitated by the dependency. In the nursing home, however, the dependency is enforced by rules, enhanced by expectations, and leads to more dependency. The perception that residents' abilities will

[193]

worsen prevents staff members from teaching residents to do more for themselves. Staff members rarely encourage residents to do things for themselves if they seem unable to do them at the outset. Nursing assistants and orderlies do their people-work duties as efficiently as possible. Rather than take the extra time to help stroke victims put on shoes one by one or help residents walk, eat, or dress, nursing assistants and orderlies do these jobs quickly. Similarly, as has been shown, the rehabilitation attempted in physical therapy loses ground to maintenance regimes on the residents' floors.

In comparing the Scottish and American nursing homes she studied, Kayser-Jones wrote: "The atmosphere of an institution and the quality of its care can either maximize one's level of functioning, thereby promoting independence; or conversely, it can minimize one's level of functioning and make one dependent upon others. At Scottsdale, for example, a portable telephone at wheelchair level can be placed in patients' rooms (every room has a telephone jack); patients can independently and privately talk with friends and relatives. But at Pacific Manor the only telephone is in the hallway at a level unreachable for those confined to wheelchairs; they must depend upon staff to dial the phone and they cannot talk privately" (1981:114). Her example illustrates how dependency is not necessarily an inevitable accompaniment to residence in the nursing home. In being expected, dependency is in part fostered by staff attitudes.

Old People as Children

People undergoing rites of passage are often likened to children because of their ignorance about the new role. Initiates are socialized into their new role by the rites. Though the residents are often characterized as children, and though they seem to be childlike initiates in a rite of passage, they are not taught.

Nor are they children, though their needs may remind staff members of children requiring care. The characterization of all old institutionalized people as children spills over from those who are the most dependent to those who may not require such extensive care. The effects of institutionalization plus the native belief that all old people are like children create pressure on the aged individuals to succumb to a self-fulfilling prophecy.[4] Treated as if he were a child, without a past, without accumulated experiences, honors, and achievements, the aged individual is reduced to his bodily ailments, which now are the sole focus of the people-work that consumes the staff members who attend to him. Kayser-Jones writes: "I propose that infantilization of the elderly occurs because staff who have no professional training and who are professionally unsure of themselves find it advantageous to establish a 'parent-child' relationship with the aged rather than an 'adult-adult' relationship. When patients are treated like children, staff do not have to take their life-long accomplishments into consideration, and they can more easily exercise their authority. Commands can be given and must be obeyed without question; patients do not participate in decisions about when to eat, take medications, and go to bed. Their absolute authority gives care-givers control and simplifies their work and routine" (1981:41).

Franklin residents are called by the diminutive versions of their names or by generic terms, such as "honey," "dearie," "sweetie," and so forth. Most employees resist the social workers' (or the residents') preference that residents be called by their surnames. The activities and events that the aged in the nursing home are supposed to enjoy are ones that children love: birthday parties are held monthly, and special outings include excursions to the zoo and the amusement park. One resident commented succinctly: "Whenever they go to the zoo, I don't bother to go. We used to live near the zoo when my children were little. I took them to the zoo every single week. I've had enough of the zoo."

Hazan describes the activities organized at the Centre similarly:

Thus, the first suggestion to boost activities amongst participants made by a new administrator introduced to the Centre was to arrange documentary and Walt Disney film shows "like they used to do in my old school." The bingo organized by outside volunteers was opened by the well-known phrase used to children "Are you sitting comfortably? Then we'll begin." On another occasion—a Sunday tea organized by outsiders—small gifts in birthday-like packets were distributed amongst those attending. A member of staff refused to join the participants in an outing to a pantomine claiming that that sort of show was only for children. An abortive attempt was made to organize an open day at the Centre to display the participants' work and activities on the implicit model of similar occasions in schools. (1980:31)

A resident described the now-defunct cooking class as follows: "I'll try anything once anyhow. They had all of us in this room. They put a bib

[195]

on each of us so we wouldn't get dirty. Then they handed each of us a bowl with two eggs in it and a spoon, and we had to mix it. And they were telling us very carefully how to do each step. Well, you can't blame them since there's so many of them in there that don't know what they're doing. The staff's only doing their job. But I'm sitting there scrambling up those eggs and I'm thinking to myself, 'What do I need this for? I've done my cake baking. If I wanted to bake a cake, what do I need to tire my arm out for? I'd do it with an automatic mixer like I used to or not at all.' Well, the class didn't work out. They stopped it." Even activities that seem intended for adults are presented as if for children. The following example comes from the music appreciation class held every week:

It's a few minutes until 10:30, and a man comes in briskly, taking off his hat and coat as he proceeds through the room. This is the music leader. He takes his place and announces himself: "Good morning. You all look very well this morning. The program is about to begin in a few minutes. Remember, there is to be no conversation during the music until 11:30. Now the curtain is about to go up." He explains that the record he is going to play is something nice and cheery to start things off since it's such a lovely spring morning. After the Mozart is over, the leader says, "Some of these records are so old they don't sound good anymore. It's like—what is it like?—it's like old bread doesn't taste good anymore. I'm going to play the next one because Max Sager requested it, and it's one of my favorites, too." In the middle of the Tchaikovsky, Sadie Berman, sitting in her wheelchair, starts talking, and people begin to shush her. The music leader gives her a long slow glare. He finally addresses himself to her companion: "Sir, sir. Should the lady be taken out? The room must be quiet. I know you understand." The man looks chastened, and nods quietly. "Tchaikovsky was very prolific. That's a word maybe two of you don't understand. He wrote a lot, a great deal of music."

Language and behaviors of the nursing-home residents are often misinterpreted. The expectation of childishness disposes staff members to react and respond in predetermined ways. Utterances from adult strangers in routine contexts are understood as reasonable, whereas neutral statements from residents lose their intended meanings, and simple behaviors framed in the nursing home environment become evidence of inabilities and childishness. A person's verbal expressions and actions are ignored, trivialized, or seem emblematic of other meanings not intended by the person. A request for something is likely to be interpreted as a complaint or considered a symptom. Requests for individualized treatment may be understood as expressions of self-centered childishness. Recall Mrs. Zeldin's enjoyment of her tomato juice. When she tells a kitchen employee that the kitchen has sent the wrong kind to her, the employee denies the charge, implying that Mrs. Zeldin has made the mistake. She is frustrated that they assume she cannot tell the difference.

The residents are not taken seriously. Stereotypes are easily applied to them. Like children, institutionalized elderly people are expected to enjoy being in one another's company automatically (Fretwell 1982). We do not expect middle-aged adults instantly to like one another but to seek out people of their choosing and to avoid people whom they dislike. The Franklin social worker did not consider that residents were silent at meals because they did not like each other (which is a prerogative of adults) or that they were avoiding quarrels (which is a strategy). Instead, residents who do not get along are regarded by many staff as childish.

Perceiving nursing home residents as children is comparable to a stripping behavior (Goffman 1961). Nonperson status is often applied to children, and similar behavior is evident in the nursing home. Adults frequently talk to one another about their children as if the children were not present. So, too, in the nursing home:

In the resident-care conference staff members are talking about a resident who is present. The resident is unable to hear what is being said because she is somewhat deaf. The resident interrupts the conversation and asks what is going on. Several staff members look surprised. In an exaggerated way, a staff member turns to face her, and speaks very slowly and loudly. After this statement, staff conversation returns to its previous quick-paced, low-decibel level.

Sometimes a social worker refers to a resident as "mother" or "dad" when talking to an adult offspring rather than as "your mother" or "your father."

Staff members may act like disagreeing and disagreeable parents who have conflicting rules and plans for the residents who seem like children. The "parents" assume that the "children" do not know what is best for them. The parents cannot agree with each other about what is best for the children. The children are dependent on parental whims and decisions. Their needs are best fulfilled when they consent to the child label associated with them and, within the definition and constraints of that label, devise strategies to pursue their goals.[5]

Retsinas disagrees with the criticism of resident infantilization and suggests that the alternatives are worse: "A formal client-provider interchange seems equally inappropriate, especially when the nursing home staff will be a surrogate family, at least in terms of time spent together, for the resident's last years. And the maternal aide at least manifests an emotional response to her patients. Many of the aides who speak so fondly of their patients also speak of them as quasi-children—not an irrational response given the dependence of the elderly person on the aide for help with the most basic tasks of daily living. While it is easy to criticize such a maternal stance, the stance bespeaks genuine affection; and in a facility where people fear dying 'emotionally alone,' that affection deserves recognition" (1986:103). While Retsinas's point is well taken, equating old people and children does not always imply affection. Too often, it is a shortcut for easy dismissal and inaccurate assumptions about the individuals.

Along with the perception that old people are like children is the denial of their sexuality. Sexual behavior, such as masturbation or residents' appreciative comments about members of the opposite sex, is often treated by staff as inappropriate, disgusting, or amusing.

Mr. Bernstein is somewhat senile, and several of the orderlies on his floor have discovered that he has a vivid interest in talking about the females that he sees. They egg him on, asking him what he thinks about this one and that one. He is specific in his appraisal of the attributes of those women he admires and of those he does not, and the orderlies listen, and giggle, and ask, "What about this one? How about her?"

In addition to the several married couples who live together in the nursing home, there are occasional amorous male-female pairs. They have limited opportunity to be discreet in the institution. Attempts to establish sexual relationships take on an adolescent quality as the couples scramble for privacy and as staff members and other residents view the relationships as illicit or ridiculous.

Residents, too, seem to think that sexual behavior in people their age is inappropriate. Some of the men described unsubtle seduction attempts by some women, which, as they related to me, they naturally rebuffed. Stanley Fierstein and his woman friend told me how they would not consider sex with each other because it was unappealing. "I don't find old women attractive," he told me later. Esther Sahlins related the following:

She was visiting the dining room of the fourth floor. She was horrified to notice that a man had his hand under the table and under a woman's dress.

When residents talk about someone's "boyfriend" or "girlfriend," it is done with a derisive edge, reminiscent of preadolescent snickering or simple jealousy.

Residents are supervised in mundane ways. For example, when a nurse dispenses medications, he or she is supposed to wait until the resident ingests the medicine to ensure that it is taken. Residents are asked each day if they have "moved their bowels."[6] Because immediate access to resident's rooms must be ensured in case of emergency, none of the doors can be locked. Individual privacy is limited, and so, necessarily, is the residents' sense of adult worth.

Decision making by residents is also hindered by the perception that residents are like children. Thus, few decisions are considered to require the resident's input since he is defined as incapable of having adult judgment. Social workers' attempts to involve residents in medical decisions are sometimes considered intrusive and irrelevant. Steinberg, Fitten, and Kachuck believe that decision making by residents is important: "The absence of any indication of doctor-patient dialogue regarding patient preferences is of concern. This is so in light of the increased vulnerability of the nursing home patient to be excluded from participation in the treatment decision-making process. This increased vulnerability is related to the special characteristics and circumstances of long-term care patients. These enhance patient passivity and dependence and tend to decrease doctor-patient interaction" (1986:362). Recognizing the difficulties of including residents in decision making, they propose a protocol for determining resident competency.[7]

Residents are rarely allowed other decision-making opportunity at Franklin. Though there is a residents' council with elected officials, it minimally influences the way the nursing home operates. It is not taken seriously by staff members or by the administration.

[199]

Staff members are discussing whether Mrs. Safrin should be allowed to continue as the council president. She has held the post for many terms, but she is increasingly unable to handle the responsibility. However, if the staff insists that she step down, she will be upset. Isn't it preferable, some staff members argue, that she remain as president, so as not to disappoint her and the residents who expect it of her?

A social worker also told me: "The residents who come to the residents' council meeting can do very little for themselves. I have to take them through all the motions, write the minutes and everything. It's not really theirs." Not permitted on committees that make policy, residents have no legitimate mechanism for changing the management. They witness changes in administration, in policy, and in staff, and their role as passive recipients remains basically the same. The care that is provided them comes at the expense of considerable independence.

Religion in the Nursing Home

While almost all the residents are Jewish, there is little attempt to make Jewishness a vital, integral part of daily life. Overall, the Judaism that exists in the nursing home consists of the Jewish identities of the individuals and the accompanying practices the residents bring with them. Whereas organizations and groups in Jewish temples brim with debate, interpretation, and strenuous preparation for holidays, fund raising, or other events, these activities are rarely seen in the nursing home. A superficial kind of Jewishness penetrates there instead.[8] The typical symbols of the holidays are used to depict the holidays, but the deeper meanings that inform them are not examined. Emblems of Jewishness, like the Star of David, a Chanukah menorah, or a typically Jewish food replace the typical Jewish vitality that reinvests significance in them.

A majority of the residents were brought up orthodox. Some have retained their orthodoxy, some have become more lax, and some have renewed religious practices after a lapse. One resident stated: "Well, we all have our ways, of course. You'd have to ask the others to know what they think. As for me, I was born in this country, but I was brought up strictly orthodox. I kept kosher for a while when I was married, but then I saw no use for it, and if I wanted to have some

[200]

bacon, why not? For me, the important thing is to keep the Ten Commandments and to be good to people; that's religion. *Traife* [non-kosher foods] doesn't matter as long as I keep the commandments." Being female, this resident was never given religious instruction, as boys traditionally were, and never learned Hebrew. Now she says she has minimal interest in attending religious services at the nursing home because she does not understand the Hebrew. Achieving the proper quorum at Franklin's daily morning service is always problematic, partly because not enough residents care to come, and partly because nurses on the floors plead insufficient staff to help needy residents get dressed and transported downstairs in time for the services.

Regardless of attendance at services, Jewishness is obvious among the residents. There are cultural factors in Judaism that bind: Yiddish expressions, jokes, and folk wisdom; common historical experiences; a religious identity; values in education and practical skills of survival; a widely shared though often argued commitment to Israel; and foods and sensory customs that have provided continuity throughout their lives. These aspects of Jewish life are maintained in some ways in the nursing home. Yiddish is heard here and there, peppering stories and providing advice and admonishment. Some residents remain involved in news events and maintain interest in Middle Eastern developments.

It is unclear whether the Jewish community has abandoned its Jewish aged or whether the nursing-home residents do not care about religion anymore. There seem to be elements of mutual disregard by both segments. In his study of elderly London Jews, Hazan reports that most of the daycare participants expressed antipathy to organizational Judaism. This sentiment originated in their feeling abandoned by the religion. Having become poor, they were unable to afford the membership costs to belong to a synagogue. They felt that the rabbis did not care about them now that they were old. They considered the teachings about reverence for the elderly to be hypocritical because of their own experiences: "Stories about ill-treatment are retailed with fury in the Centre. One participant claimed that he was virtually expelled from a synagogue on the Day of Atonement as a non-member of the congregation. Another described how he was snubbed by the warden of his synagogue because he had been in arrears with his bills. One experience particularly incensed the participants. It was the allegation of a man confined to a wheelchair that he was refused admission

[201]

to his own synagogue on a Saturday, not because there were no adequate facilities to accommodate him, but because the Rabbi defined the wheelchair as a vehicle breaching the law against using transport on the Sabbath" (1980:101–2). These elderly Jews rejected their old congregations in return, and believed that they practiced their Judaism in their relationships with another by helping one another.

Few of the Franklin staff members are Jewish. Virtually no one on the staff understands or can speak Yiddish except for an expression or two.[9] When staff members know a few words of Yiddish, they often use the words for instant rapport:

One of the residents offers the nurse a piece of chocolate he has received from his granddaughter."Do I look like I need that?" laughs the nurse, trying to say no. "Just look at that tuchas" *[rear end].*

Even such knowledge of Yiddish is rare. Bernice Meyerhov has a good relationship with her nursing assistant because Mrs. Meyerhov speaks Spanish, not because her nursing assistant knows Yiddish. Ignorance of Jewish customs and religious holidays and beliefs is almost universal among the staff. Anecdotes about anti-Semitic attitudes among employees were related to me, and misunderstandings about Jewish beliefs and customs are not rare.

Today is the beginning of Tisha B'Av, the commemoration of the destruction of the Second Temple. Helen Scarborough and Lil Sullivan ask a couple of social workers if either of them is Jewish. Helen and Lil have to read a script that a Jewish member of the staff has prepared (on her own time) for the religious and historical significance of the holiday. Helen and Lil need help about the pronunciation of various words. One word is "pogrom." After being told the correct pronunciation, they ask what the word means. With amazement the social workers tell Helen and Lil what the pogroms in Russia were. It is significant that Helen has always told everyone that she loves history. She has worked in this nursing home for a few years, claims that she enjoys talking with the residents about their pasts, yet does not know about the infamous raids on Jews in Russia at the turn of the century. Many of the current residents are survivors of the pogroms and remember them vividly.

Social workers, some of whom are Jewish, have overheard derisive comments from nursing assistants and orderlies, such as: "She's just a bitchy Jewish old lady." Other staff members seem more fascinated with the "strangeness" of certain Jewish customs: "If you really want to see something, come in here early in the morning when they're putting on all those whatchamacallits. Don't try to disturb them then; that's when they pray." Not all Jewish holidays and commemorations, such as Israel Independence Day, are celebrated. Ignorance of or antipathy to Jewish history and culture may be the reasons. Lisa, a Jewish staff member, remarked about the clambakes at Franklin. (Shellfish is a category of food never eaten by Jews who observe *Kashrut*, the kosher rules.) One was scheduled on a Jewish holiday. She has also overheard anti-Semitic remarks about and to the residents.

Another problem in observing Jewish rituals involves rivalries among residents. Certain individuals are said to monopolize ritually important tasks. But when honors are more fairly divided, there are complaints that the rituals are not performed properly.

When Ida Kanter was admitted, she noticed that there were no Friday evening candle-lighting ceremonies. The social worker suggested that the resident organize it. Mrs. Kanter remembers to procure the candlesticks, to put on a white tablecloth, and to have wine glasses and wine available for the occasions. However, the fact that she is de facto in charge of the Shabbos candle ritual has made her the target of other residents who resent her position of assumed authority.

While staff members have little or no background in matters Jewish, occasionally, a flicker of information about Jewish history or culture is exploited by the staff as the "explanation" of some heretofore baffling resident behavior. The fact that Jews were in concentration camps during World War II completely "explains" any reluctance by residents to wear identification bracelets now. However, these shortcuts to cultural and personal understanding rarely penetrate beyond, or dissuade staff members from, their original preconceptions. Because residents are not asked "how things were" or what meaning something has, staff members' beliefs about the residents need not be challenged nor revised. Furthermore, as has been noted, the residents themselves do not go into these issues, but shy away from discussions of all sorts. The fervent debate that Myerhoff (1979) described among the

[203]

Jews in the senior center does not on here. Thus, there is no pertinent material from which newly meaningful forms of old ritual can spring. Instead, the "chicken soup" Judaism of the nursing home acts as a thin reminder of the real thing and fails to provide viable answers and to heal.

The Unanswerable Questions

Many of the residents have endured difficult lives and have been unable to devise satisfactory answers to the plaguing question "Why me?" The setting of the nursing home offers no solace even though some of the residents are bound together by similar experiences. For example, some of the children of the residents have married non-Jews or have divorced. They have no good explanation for these events. In telling about such catastrophes as divorce and intermarriage in the family, some residents shrug and do not attempt to explain.

Mr. Sager was telling me about his wonderful daughter-in-law, who is not Jewish but is nice. Mr. Sager has changed his mind about intermarriage accordingly. Even though his son has died and the daughter-in-law has moved thousands of miles away, she telephones him, sends him letters, and never forgets his birthday. He is touched by her thoughtfulness.

More battling and no less disturbing is the fact that numerous residents have outlived their children. The death of a child is considered a particularly harsh tragedy. Many of the residents consider themselves too old still to be living; it seems a cruel joke that a son or daughter with children still in college or graduate school should die from cancer or in a car accident or by a sudden heart attack. As Moore has written about the Chagga of Kilamanjaro, people expect an orderly timing about the succession of deaths: "Over the course of life, men see themselves moving place by place up the seniority ladder of the lineage. It is clear who is *due* to die next and who is to succeed him. When people die out of turn, that is something to be explained. It means that something has gone wrong in the order of things, and there may be witchcraft or curses to reckon with" (1978:31).

At the nursing home, people struggle for explanations to satisfy, but rarely succeed. Mr. Sager looks baffled as he describes how his perfectly healthy son "just died" one day at age 50. There is too much that does not make sense: it does not make sense to continue a strange, day-to-day life in a nursing home for month after month and year after year, when one seems to oneself to be far past an appropriate time to die. It does not make sense that an adult child should die while his aged parent lives on in this way. One resident said, "Every day I am surprised to wake up. 'Why didn't you take me last night, God?' I always ask him." For most, it seems the inexplicability of these things must remain the "answer": "Never think," counsels a resident, "that you know what is going to happen. Just enjoy your marriage, your husband, and your children. You never know. My Sam had a bad heart, and yet, thank God, he lived until he was 85. You see?" Residents do not have a ritualized or formal opportunity to discuss these inexplicable tragedies with one another. They may not know that they are not the only ones who have experienced these losses. Ritual, religion, and the companionship of caring others would help.

No Ritual, No Communitas

The lack of ritual makes the passage of each individual through the nursing home an isolated struggle. Each resident enters Franklin alone, and each one finds his own way of adapting to the ways of the institution alone. The staff members and the Harrison community do little to encourage the residents to find ties among themselves. Though the residents share Jewishness, heritage, jokes, customs, and much of the same history, they eschew their commonalities and seem to find more solace in their isolation.

The silence regarding death may be due to an orthodox prohibition restricting talk about death, though other Jewish nursing homes manage to include death counseling in their regimens. It may also be due to death anxiety.[10] The lack of discussion of, and preparation for, death contrasts sharply with the hospice approach. Active preparation for, and acknowledgement of, death in the nursing home might well foster the development of transition-easing rituals, which in turn would foster the development of group solidarity and communitas. Rejecting talk of death, however, prevents preparation and rituals from occurring.

Hochschild discusses how the elderly widows of Merrill Court constructed a ritual for a woman who had died:

[205]

Immediately the community held an emergency meeting to arrange for the funeral supper. The flower committee ordered a $15 wreath and many volunteered to cook a dish for the bereaved relatives. A cold supper was arranged for thirty-five relatives and friends. Nearly everyone in the community went to view the body at a local funeral parlor, to the funeral service, and to the burial. In the following week there was a moratorium on work, as became the custom with deaths in the building. These customs gave those left a chance to cry, to express sorrow, to comfort, and to be comforted without fear of embarrassment; and it gave them a chance to *do* something—call people, buy flowers, bake pies. In this way the community taught itself about death. Although they were part of a collectivity that was itself immortal and in which the deceased were replaced, they each realized their own mortality. In going to the funerals of others, it is as if they were experimentally going to their own. (1973:80–81)

An example of a "bungled" death, in contrast, was reported by Keith as follows:

The first death in the residence occurred at night, and the director tried to minimize what he thought would be its depressing effect on other residents by giving it no formal recognition. No announcement was made in the dining hall; no plans were made for residents to participate in a funeral service; no one was informed of the time the hearse would arrive. . . . The dining room, the hallways, and the lobby were agitated that evening. "I don't want that to happen to me," several people told me—"that" not being death, they specified, but a bungled, undignified funeral. The anxiety tinged with disappointment which permeated that day brings to light two basic facts about rituals. First, in a very profound sense, they give people something to do; and second, they are also, quite simply, important events. . . . Those who are left behind need something to do precisely because in a deeper sense there is nothing they can do. . . . People had, after all, been cheated out of a major event because something as important as a death had gone unmarked. (1982b:98–100)

As a result of this incident, the community members presented a formal request that announcements of deaths be made in the future. The community members used the incident to create a procedure by which they would mark new deaths among them. In this way they fashioned a ritual that clarified their bonds with each other and that explained to themselves their nearness to death. They made an event that connected them to the deceased and to each other. It provided comfort, asserted that continuity was important and would be maintained, and assured each individual a role and a place within this and similar rituals. They had created communitas.

Both Keith and Hochschild stress how "doing something" is a crucial part of ritual. Their emphasis is important in part because it underscores the significance of reciprocity for making meaning. Reciprocity is acting for something, contributing toward a goal. Doing something that is considered worthwhile contrasts with the makework, time-filling aspect of activities found in nursing homes and other total institutions. In the rituals described by Keith and Hochschild, doing something meant putting meaning into action with others similarly positioned. The people in both situations were doing something for themselves and for one another.

Victor Turner did not believe that communitas was always present in liminal states. He maintained that there were restrictive conditions in which communitas would surface: "I am suggesting that this process only works where there is already a high level of communitas in the society that performs the ritual, the sense that a basic generic bond is recognized beneath all its hierarchical and segmentary differences and oppositions. Communitas in ritual can only be evoked easily when there are many occasions outside the ritual on which communitas has been achieved" (1974:56). This passage strictly qualifies the presence of communitas in ritual and helps to explain how in rite-of-passage situations in which liminality is clearly present, communitas need not be. Such is the case of the Franklin Nursing Home: while existence is liminal, there is more isolation than communitas. Instead of communitas, residents stay by themselves and try to be "good" patients. Rather than find similarities among themselves to bind them together, residents emphasize and maintain their differences. Instead of creating the exuberance found in communitas, residents often distrust one another, compete with one another, and denigrate one another. Except for the outstanding exception of the work and camaraderie in physical therapy, there are no difficult tasks to undergo, and there seems little reason for the residents to bond together, little reason to help one another and to reciprocate. While acknowledging that they share a similar fate, while knowing that they all suffer from not having alternatives available outside the nursing home, while speaking about common Jewish customs, histories, and holidays, they share little. Instead of the harrowing transition in most rites of passage worldwide, the transition in the nursing home is thought by staff to be protected

[207]

and tame. As if separated from the ongoing rigors of life and from the deteriorating course of the body, the residents wait.

The illusion of timelessness belies the certainty of how limited the residents' time actually is. The time of future peril that intact residents perceive as their fate threatens the quality of resident relationships rather than intensifies them. The residents interact superficially and guardedly. There can be little chance of communitas where the present is benignly misrepresented as safe and timeless, the future is known to be uncertain and perilous, and individuals serve as reminders to one another of their present fragile security and future certain danger.

Communitas need not be prevented by the fact that new nursing-home residents make their admission to the nursing home separately. Though the timing of each entrance is individual, communitas could still be generated by rituals articulating the commonalities among the initiates once installed in the nursing home. Working together in physical therapy, for example, forges a solidarity unique within the nursing home. Similarly, the deaths described by Hochschild and Keith triggered rituals that made explicit how the members of the group were alike. Without such rituals, the threat was that they remain separate in the vulnerable time of mourning.

If, as in other rites of passage, there were rituals at the Franklin Nursing Home that served to explain and cushion the participants' situation, there would likely be more communitas and shared identification. However, staff members disagree about goals for the residents and perceive no reason for preparation or teaching for the next stage. Staff members splinter among themselves, and residents do likewise. Instead of adapting bits and pieces of old ritual to novel crises and conflicts as in the senior center Myerhoff described (1979), Franklin residents lack the means to create ritual and communitas, and loneliness is left. Instead of the Jewish community joining together to forge a new integration of past values, present experiences, and common anticipations about the future with the residents, it gives custodial care.

Finally, with the major exception of physical therapy, nursing-home liminality contains no tasks that residents must fulfill. Whereas learning and trials are the initiate's ticket to gaining admission to the next phase or status in most rites of passage, nothing is expected of nursing-home residents in their passage. This nonreciprocity makes them ineligible for serious treatment as adult persons. Residence at Franklin is a liminal state without communitas because it is a timeless state that merely ends when it ends. In other transitions, individuals can look forward to a new status in which certain behaviors, activities, and prestige will be expected of them; residents in the nursing home are forever recipients. No requirement for reciprocity and little incentive for exchange join death denial and the conflict of staff members to form a gruesome liminality. By equating the aged with children, staff members transform the threat of death into the familiarity of nurturance. The overwhelming needs of these aged individuals can be more easily manipulated by nurturing mother figures than by health professionals attempting to assuage the complaints and ailments of adults who are like them, only older and physically more helpless. In this way, the nursing-home residents are made both unthreateningly familiar, as children, and distantly "other." When nursing-home residents can be perceived as a separate and alien category, staff members are relieved of identification with them. The danger inherent in the liminality is thus contained, and the liminality remains unresolved.

Notebook:
Resident-Care Conference

Dr. Corning has just arrived. Gladys, a social worker, presents the first resident, Clara Singer, 85, who was born in a nearby city, one of five children. She worked in a hat factory until retirement. Her husband died years ago of a heart ailment. They had one son and four grandchildren, who live out of state. A sister, Bernice Adler, lives at Franklin; another sister, with whom Mrs. Singer had lived, died several years ago. Her father had owned an umbrella business.

Three and a half years ago after falling from bed, she said, "I'm sick and need to be taken care of," and was admitted. She has little contact with family members. The other residents tolerate her, though her anxiety bothers many of them. She shows concern for them, however. On the Goldfarb mental status exam she scored five out of ten, but it isn't clear how much anxiety contributed to her low score. She attends the large parties at the nursing home with her sister, and the two of them visit each other often. Mrs. Singer used to do fine needlework but has given it up. The staff thinks she should be encouraged to do more of it. A social worker, Fran, says that she is one of the most anxious residents in the home. Her medical problems are listed on the board by a nurse as follows: herniated disc disease, diabetes, personality disorder, anxiety neurosis, arteriosclerotic heart disease, and memory loss.

She was the subject of the medical student conference last Wednesday. Attending two meetings in one week has exacerbated her anxiety. Gladys says she wishes such meetings were planned better; she just found out about last week's meeting. She reports that Mrs. Singer is so nervous that she has bitten every one of her nails.

While the staff is talking, a large man comes in awkwardly, and sits down. He explains that he's here for the conference on Mrs. Singer, his mother. Dr. Corning says they are still discussing her, but he can stay. He asks the man if a psychiatrist has seen his mother. No. The son says that the Franklin Nursing Home has done wonders for his mother. When Gladys asks him if his mother has always been so anxious, he laughs and says yes. In answer to whether it's an anxious family, he says most of them are, except for one of Mrs. Singer's sisters. Gladys thinks that Mrs. Singer needs more reassurance.

This comment prompts the staff to discuss how nasty many of the residents in the wing are. A social worker says they are jealous of each other, and they make cruel remarks when someone shows affection. One nurse thinks they are snobs. Gloria and Jean think this behavior has to do with their fear that they will become dependent.

Back to the son. He thinks his mother is doing quite well, but he cannot tolerate her visits at home: she drives him nuts. "She has a cheese sandwich and then gets back on the phone asking when can she come back to the home." The nurse concurs with the son's assessment.

Mrs. Singer is asked to come in. Dr. Corning takes her hands, leans forward, and says that he's so sorry that he didn't realize that she had been in another conference so recently. He tells her not to worry about it; everyone thinks that she is doing just fine. She says that that's nice to hear and wants to know what everyone thinks of her. When Dr. Corning responds that everyone thinks she is very nice, she is glad to hear this. The son comments that she is always concerned about what others think. Gloria asks her if she is going to help them out with needlework. Mrs. Singer says she will try, but her eyes bother her. Dr. Corning checks her chart to see when she last had an eye appointment. He finds that it was about six months ago.

He says that she can go. As she is leaving she turns to her son and asks if he is coming; he says he's staying for a few minutes and then he'll be leaving; she repeats what he said and asks if it's all right if she calls him around 4:30, and he says that that's fine. After she leaves, the son says that she calls him every day at 9:00 and at 4:30. The staff asks if that has changed, and he says that she used to call him erratically, and now it is regular. Gladys asks Dr. Corning if Mrs. Singer should be given a drug for anxiety, but he wants to try nonmedication remedies instead, such as reassurance or activities. The son now leaves, thanking the staff for all they're doing and again repeats that coming here is the best thing that ever happened to her.

[211]

The next resident to be presented is Evelyn Tischler. The social worker says she is 89 years old and she and her son have had a very difficult relationship. She was admitted three years ago for several months. While she was here, she was adamant about returning to the community, and she did. Now she is back because her eyesight has become so bad that she is unable to remain in her apartment alone. The social worker explains that the doctor has discussed the possibility of surgery to remove the cataract. The son is determined that his mother not have surgery. He is certain she is against it also, and he wishes to spare her. He is furthermore concerned that his mother wants to make this stay a temporary one again, like the last time, but he knows that this is her last stop. He does not dare discuss this with her. He tells all of us that she is not a woman who can be crossed. Before Mrs. Tischler comes in, the staff and the son discuss whether the surgery is feasible or not. It seems that she has made a fairly good adjustment in the nursing home, and she is able to get around quite well. The surgery is more straightforward than the son was originally led to believe, and it is likely to have dramatically beneficial results. Nonetheless, the son insists that he knows his mother, and he will never consent to her surgery. Dr. Corning repeats that surgery may not be necessary, considering her adaptation, but because it is simpler than expected, it may be something his mother desires. "Remember," Dr. Corning cautions, "your mother is entirely competent to make her own decision in the matter. This will be her decision, not yours," he finishes, carefully.

The mother is asked to come in. Dr. Corning introduces himself and Mrs. Tischler remembers him immediately. "I'll never forget the time," she says laughing, "when I was in your office, and you yelled at me, 'Don't waste my valuable time!' because I didn't want to do what you wanted me to do!" She seems to cherish the memory, and Dr. Corning and the rest of us are laughing, too. She holds his arm roughly and strongly. He asks defensively, "Have you forgiven me yet, Evelyn?" and she says immediately, "No!" "But Evelyn, that was years ago. I'm not so set in my ways anymore; I've gotten better—haven't I, Mrs. Rubin?" he asks the social worker, who backs him up by saying, "Yes, he has, Mrs. Tischler; he has gotten better with age." Mrs. Tischler laughs appreciatively and says again how she'll never forget that day.

Now Dr. Corning leans very close to her and signals a serious tone. "Mrs. Tischler," he says solemnly, "I have to ask you something today. When you were admitted this time, who made the decision to come *here?" She answers quickly that it was her decision. "Do you think it was a good decision?" he asks her carefully. She answers immediately that it was the right decision because she couldn't manage by herself anymore. Now, he asks, "Do you think you are going to leave here or are you staying?" "Oh, there's no question about that," she responds without hesitation. "I have to stay here. I've already given notice that my apartment should be closed up. My son will take care of that." As she speaks, the son's face is transformed; he looks astonished and relieved.*

The social worker whispers to Dr. Corning that he should ask about the surgery. He waves her question away, saying he does not want to ask that, but then he asks it. He says that her physician is pleased to see that she has adjusted very well to the new setting and that she has managed to get around the nursing home quite well. Gingerly, he continues: there is some question that cataract surgery could be performed quite easily and might help her become more independent than she already is. If that were her physician's recommendation, and she and he reviewed all the risks and benefits to the surgery, what might she say? "Well," Mrs. Tischler answers slowly, "I might want to go along with it and do it then if that was the case." Again, the son's jaw drops. Dr. Corning continues, "It's my job to give you all the facts and to make recommendations because you can't make decisions without all the facts, right, Mrs. Tischler?" She says yes and again grabs his arm, pinches his cheek vigorously, and repeats the story about his long-ago anger in his office. Dr. Corning and Mrs. Tischler look like they thoroughly enjoy one another. After she leaves with her nursing assistant, the social workers compliment him on a job well done. The son looks happy and relieved. With modesty and pleasure, Dr. Corning says that when this meeting works it's because the family members and the resident are genuinely part of the group decision-making process. He looks as if he could crow.

[10]

Summary and Conclusion

Life for the aged in nursing homes is often presented as dreary, sad, and lonely. Many accounts document abuse and fraud, and these findings are indisputable. Cross-cultural evidence about the aged illuminates both the similarities and the differences between the United States and other cultures and shows that many of the aged do not consider themselves unfortunate, abused, or victimized, but continue living in varied and worthwhile ways.

This study of the Franklin Nursing Home offers a mixed view. A well-thought-of nursing home, Franklin offers many good services. Many of the residents express satisfaction at being there and actively chose to be admitted, and many staff members demonstrate sensitive and caring qualities. On the other hand, this institution shares with others the problems of insensitive and ambivalent treatment of the aged.

Three main theoretical threads have been emphasized in this account. One describes the contribution of Goffman's salient description of total institutions and how his treatment illuminates the behaviors and attitudes of those at Franklin. But whereas Goffman described how total institutions function, his treatment fails to explain much of the behavior and care management found in the nursing home. Elucidating how his description is apt as well as defining its limitations allowed me to explore the dual effect of nonreciprocity and liminality without communitas. A resident of the nursing home is a recipient whose obligation to repay is deemed both unnecessary and impossible. Because he cannot contribute, he is perceived as closer to nature (that is, death) than to culture (life), and his status as a human is devalued (Amoss 1981). This nonreciprocal status links with the third factor, the liminality of his transition in the rite of passage. Together they increase the isolation, neediness, and passivity of the old people in the nursing home and make them appear to be like the children the staff members say they are. This potent combination creates the problem of nursing-home residence.

The ability to give, receive, and repay seems to be so basic to human social life that it is often the crucial mark of personhood. The inability to repay, on the other hand, is often a criterion of not being a "real" person. In the United States being a recipient is ambivalently perceived both as a right and as a stigma. Status as a recipient is linked to being dependent, and being dependent in turn is associated with nonresponsible, nonautonomous, childlike status.

The home-versus-hospital dichotomy that underlies the lifeways of the institution, reflecting divisions in staff ideologies and preventing staff and resident cohesion, connects the ideas of reciprocity and liminality. Notions associated with the home idea have to do with community, purpose, connectedness, and comfort. Members of a well-functioning home work together, assert their allegiance to one another, and rearticulate in new forms and contexts how they are meaningful to one another. In the hospital, on the other hand, patients are sick, receive care by staff members, and comply with staff orders. Patients need not communicate with one another; their primary relationship is with the doctor and the other staff members ministering to them individually. Further, they need not be active in getting well. Home principles in this analogy therefore translate into community and reciprocity, and hospital principles correspond to isolation, passivity, and nonreciprocity. In the nursing home there is evidence of community and reciprocity when home factors come to the fore. These are the times when staff members and residents act like friends, when residents demonstrate support for one another by helping out, and when residents work together in physical therapy to improve their condition.

I have defined entrance to the nursing home as a rite of passage with few if any rituals. The entrance is lonely, accomplished primarily by a series of leave-takings from a past life. The resident makes the adjustment alone; it is accomplished without institutional, community, or ritual assistance.

By and large, residents of the nursing home are "protected" from knowledge about diseases and disabilities in old age, and the subject of death is avoided by staff members. There is no consensus about goals, little sharing and cooperation, and no one definition of what entrance to the nursing home means among staff members. Without sharing and without ritual, the individual old people endure the solitary passage en masse.

The liminality described here is different from that described by Victor Turner because individuals make the passage separately and because there is no communitas in this nursing home. The lack of communitas is due to the fact that there is no solidarity about the nursing-home experience, there is little community involvement, and there are no clear expectations or rules about how residents should make the passage. Many have entered the nursing home because alternative supports in the community were not available, and they must be dependent and passive. Some maximize their deficits as a strategy: they have swapped their roles as autonomous adults for the security the nursing home offers, and they seem to have happily let go of their burdensome responsibilities. For others, however, even the good nursing home represents an intolerable life, and they wish for death. They are "decultured" and brought closer to nature, treated like problem-filled bodies that must be serviced and maintained, separated from their owners, who are not permitted a say in their care and use. They are misunderstood as children, as persons with no pasts, as recipients with no legitimate input into the factors that determine their lives. Treated alike by the staff, they recognize no bonds with each other—instead they splinter into their heterogeneous identities because there are no rituals to bind them together as separate individuals undergoing the passage from life in the community to death. The poignant exception to this inexorable process is the ritual-like drama played out everyday in the physical therapy setting. It is more poignant because of its singularity in the nursing-home experience. Here people are most themselves, in all their individuality, but at the same time, they strive together against odds of failure to buoy themselves and one another in their agonizing quest for physical mastery. Individuality is cherished here as well as transcended in service to the group work effort. [1]

Though residents in nursing homes must exhibit some competence in order to make decisions and be allowed control, autonomy and confidence are undermined in dependency-fostering situations. When the aged are defined as a problem, as a conglomeration of deficits, the incompetent status of the group is achieved. As Estes (1979) has

[216]

shown, the social welfare programs that have been constructed around the idea of aging as a problem perpetuate the problem. Medicare and Medicaid regulations operating within Franklin and upon which the nursing home is entirely dependent ensure that nonperson people-work treatment of residents by staff is favored over more humane considerations. These hospital principles ensure that life-prolonging measures prevail, and they guarantee that choice and control be located in staff members and in outside agencies that determine the rules and provide the monetary blood that keeps the institution alive.

These factors create difficult nursing-home living: Federal and state rules restrict competent residents from doing more for themselves and for the more dependent residents. Nursing-home admission is the last stage before death; yet staff members differ in whether they help prepare individuals for death or whether they retreat from such preparations. Social and emotional supports decrease while body-preserving mechanisms are maintained. People-work jobs determine the quality of staff-resident relationships, devaluing both the employees and the old people. The healing and explanatory roles of religion are missing from nursing home life. Community members prop up the nursing home financially, but retreat from personal, sustained involvement with the residents within. The institution develops ways to have self-sufficient services in the nursing home and thereby deepens the separation between itself and the community. These factors are powerful ones that residents cannot fight.

Toward Mourning and Memory

Gerontologists of different theoretical backgrounds and persuasions have issued recommendations for the improvement of nursing-home residence overall. Recommendations that would minimize the institutional nature of the long-term-care setting by involving community members and by enabling more resident control and input into the institution would seem appropriate. Barney (1987), for example, has suggested the advantages of community involvement in nursing homes. When community councils are organized, residents, family members, and staff members share information to effect practical and relevant improvements in the nursing home. The volunteer program at Franklin could be strengthened, and volunteers could be encouraged to interact directly with residents whenever possible. Residents could be encouraged to help with fund raising. They could help sell the items they make in recreational therapy. The residents' council could be strengthened and allowed more decision-making power.

Fostering religious practice and conducting educational or support groups concerned with aging are examples of principles that might mitigate the liminality of nursing-home residence. Residents and family members could be educated about the aging process so that they would not be terrified that what they see happen to others is inevitable for them. Family members could be involved in groups with residents to ease adjustment to the nursing home, alleviate family guilt about the need for institutionalization, and provide a forum for airing some of these issues. Religious leaders could be urged to participate more actively. The most capable residents could be encouraged to speak to temple groups in the community. Residents could teach Yiddish to children in the local Hebrew schools. Yiddish could be taught to nursing assistants and orderlies. Berman, Weiner, and Fishman (1986) found an enthusiastic staff response to a Yiddish program at a Jewish home for the aged and believe that sensitivity to the residents was increased in the process. Volunteers from the community could tape the oral histories of willing residents. These could be made into a book and sold to raise money for the nursing home. The staff could be taught Jewish history and the basics of Jewish belief and custom. Residents could be addressed by the names they prefer. These are just a few examples of simple things that could be done.

In all, benefits might come from expecting the more competent residents to maintain ties to the community and to contribute services to the nursing home and Harrison whenever possible. The more able aged should be expected to give as well as to receive. In whatever ways possible, the responsible, reciprocating capabilities of the aged should be fostered and encouraged.

In short, nursing-home residence might be considerably improved if steps were taken to remedy the two main problems: (1) increase the strengths of the residents in order to enhance their independence, and (2) create community rituals to provide cohesion and solidarity, which aid the transition in the rite of passage. People need to "do something" in order to feel worthwhile and count as human beings. They especially need to "do something" in this more secular age when they are encountering the deaths of others and preparing to die themselves. Myerhoff writes: "There is every reason to believe that rites of passage are as important now as they have always been, for our social and psychological well-being. Indeed, given the fragmented, confusing, complex, and disorderly nature of modern experience, perhaps they are more important: to orient and motivate us in the predictable and unique life crises that present themselves. But now we are left to devise for ourselves the myths, rituals, and symbols needed to endow life with clarity and significance; we do so alone, often in ignorance and always in uncertainty. Our needs have not changed, though the gods, demons, heroes, and spirits that once animated our ceremonies have fallen into disuse" (1982:129). As was shown in the last chapter, the French retirees described by Keith and the widows of Merrill Court described by Hochschild took ritual making into their own hands and did something together about the life crises they were individually and collectively facing.

Other nursing homes manage to allow residents more say in their care. The Jewish nursing home in which residents raise monies and sometimes work in local businesses is a prime example of utilizing the capacities of intact residents. Another Jewish nursing home has confronted the issue of death ritual by employing a Jewish chaplain trained in counseling. When a resident dies, a memorial service is always held on the premises of the nursing home. It benefits residents, relatives, and staff members, and it serves as an explicit mark that the resident lived in the nursing home, and died there, leaving mourners and memories. The nursing home has also started a bereavement program in which the survivors, including family members as well as residents and staff members who were attached to the deceased, are encouraged to seek group support (Kronenberg 1983).

Myerhoff wrote that rituals can be fashioned where none currently exist: "Menopause, surgery, 'empty nests,' retirement, are all regular occasions in life that go largely uncelebrated. All those can be opportunities for rites of passage, transformed from traumatic experiences or disorienting lonely episodes into commemorations that acknowledge change. The spontaneous ritual acts that we so often do alone—burning an unfaithful lover's photographs or returning gifts from one no longer cherished, the cutting of hair or cleaning house to announce to oneself that a new phase of life is beginning—all these are nascent rites of passage that can be enlarged, formalized, made to include important people, memorialized with objects, notes, or records that are kept in recognition that the transition was successfully accomplished" (1982:132). Given the vast wealth of ritual material to which the residents of Franklin have access by dint of their long Jewish lives, it seems likely that relevant new rituals could be created with the help of an accommodating staff and interested community and family members.

The fact that each individual enters the nursing home at a different time need not be a deterrent to the presence of ritual or to the development of communitas in the rite of passage. Ritual forms of welcome and socialization could be fashioned to take each new resident from his former status outside the institution to his new one inside. Communitas might develop because residents have the entrance experience to talk about, one they discover others have shared. Ceremonies could be devised to welcome the new residents who enter the nursing home each month. Those who have been in the nursing home for more than one month might be given instrumental roles in this welcoming ritual in recognition of their having passed through the rigors of entrance already. The separateness of individuals could be maintained at the same time that their commonality is celebrated.

The emotional and cultural gulf separating the Franklin Nursing Home from the Harrison community could and should be bridged. Perhaps the easiest route would begin with initiatives from the nursing home. Family members and others from Harrison could be invited to the nursing home to participate in educational or festive occasions that would help shrink the gap between them. If the Jewish community of Harrison made more of a concerted effort to be involved in the nursing home, the aged individuals among them might not be perceived as scary and alien. Fear and distaste too often prevent younger people from acknowledging that they will one day be old, made dependent, choiceless, and receiving. The very first steps come from our understanding that the old people are "us" eventually, that there is continuity between the ages, and that dependency and independence recur throughout the life cycle. In recognizing these links, perhaps we all have a future.

Voice:
Priscilla Frails, Nursing Assistant

Well, I have been a nursing assistant for fifteen years, and it has been and still is a joy and pleasure working with the elderly and taking care of them. It is rewarding, and it's a privilege. I feel that in order to be a dedicated and devoted nursing assistant, you must maintain infinite love—because without love for the work this is the wrong profession for you. I'm nervous! I don't know why I'm nervous. I'm usually very comfortable with you in our conversations. But I guess because of the tape recorder. . . .

I have a special love in my heart for my work. I love taking care of the elderly. It gives me inner joy to be able to take care of their needs and do the things that they're not able to do for themselves. They tell me many many times that when I'm not there, it's a big difference. And when I'm there, they feel very secure. I take time with them. I take time to listen. Regardless of how busy I am, I give them a few moments. "I'm so happy to see you," they will say. "It's so wonderful that you are here today." When I'm not there, I'm deeply missed. It gives me such satisfaction to know that they really miss me when I'm not there.

You really have to have a compassionate heart. If you're not humble and if you're a very high-strung person, you're not able to relate. Suppose they're trying to tell you something or explain something and you just don't have the time to listen, you know? I feel you have to be very understanding and listen to their complaints. When they come here, they have to adjust, and it's very difficult for them. Some never adjust to the institution. And some of them really die with a broken heart.

[221]

You know what I do? I talk with them spiritually. I let them know that God loves them, and I tell them to take one day at a time and accomplish what they can in that day, and tomorrow will be a brighter day for them. It's very difficult for them to accept this place as their home. Some of them want to come. They feel that if they stay with their children they will be a burden to their children. But the ones who don't come on their own—some of them feel very depressed over it.

I always give them an encouraging word and say they'll feel happier if they'll only learn to accept. I tell them, "You know, just count your blessings. Even though you're here, you still have a lot to be thankful for." And then I tell them, "You're able to do this for yourself; you're able to do that," and they really begin to see what they're able to accomplish for themselves, and this gives them a desire to go to the different activities and to participate.

When they come here, I tell them to do as much as they can and what they are not able to do, then I will do for them. Some try and some don't. If they don't do it, I continue to encourage them, and I do it [laughs]. But I don't force. If they say they just can't do it, then I just do it. I accept it.

It is a joy to work with someone who is appreciative. You go into her room and she has a smile on her face. It just makes your whole day. It's a pleasure to work with them and to care for them and to just help them. That sort of person is not demanding; they're very patient. Supposing I was doing something for someone else, right? And I would tell this individual just to wait a moment. And he says, "Okay, whenever you can come." Whereas if it's a person that's very demanding, very impatient, you say, "Wait just a moment," and then you get verbally abused. Yes. Usually I will correct a person and tell them, "You have to have patience. I'm here to help you, not to fight with you. I'm here to do what I can, but I'm not here to be abused." I'm a person. I have respect for the elderly. I treat them with love and dignity, and I want to be treated with respect. So when I do have someone like this, obnoxious, very demanding, or can't wait or just really arrogant—what I do: I inform the nurse and then the nurse informs the social service, and then the resident gets lectured about it.

The other day, Friday, I had already served the lunch, and I had given everybody coffee, so this person wanted a second cup of coffee. So I went over to the container, and of all times, it was empty. So I said, "I can make a Sanka for you." Just by saying, "I would make a

Sanka for you," he starts screaming and yelling, "I don't want that Sanka! Every time I ask for a second cup of coffee, why can't I get it?" as though I was the fault of that, you know. But I was willing to make him another cup of coffee [laughs]. So I kept silent and then I informed the nurse and the social worker and they talked with him. So this is the only way you can handle a person like this with an attitude like this. It's as though he's angry with the world, you know. Regardless of what you do, he's not pleased. Very, very difficult.

My job can be very stressful, frustrating at times. I find especially so when we are understaffed. When there are three nurses in the wing, three nursing assistants, it's really beautiful. Because you have even extra time to spend with them. A lot of times they just want to express themselves and how they feel inside. A lot of times when I go in to make their bed or just go in to say hello to them, they want you to sit down. They want to talk to you for a few minutes. So when we are fully staffed, you are able to do that. You are able to do extra things for them. But when you're understaffed, the work load is tremendous. It's just tremendous. When I go home, I feel good in my heart, but my body physically is just exhausted.

A lot of times you learn about their families and many trials and tribulations that they went through, and how God blessed them and gave them the courage to continue to press forward. I say to myself, "Oh. God did this for you. I know He could do the same for me if I had to go through a similar experience." And then they tell you about their country and how they lived and what they went through, and how they themselves were enriched, how they were strengthened through all the trials they went through.

If the nursing homes could just have more help, it would just be so wonderful. That would eliminate so many problems. It would. And then we could spend more time with the residents. Especially in the summer. In the spring and summer, I like to take my residents outside and be with them, and a lot of times when we're understaffed we can't do that.

I give baths. I do TPRs—which is temp, respiration, and pulse. I take blood pressures, I do weights, I have to serve two meals. Footcare, handcare. Make sure that their nails are cleaned and trimmed. I like to soak their feet because it's so refreshing—they love it. Yes. And while I'm soaking their feet, then we have a chance to chat, you know? So that's very enjoyable. It's wonderful. We can't do it every day. Sometimes they give us an extra girl, but when we don't get the extra

*girl on, I just do the major things. And a lot of times on my weekend
on, I will give them their footcare because it's not as busy as during
the weekday.*

*Even though we're understaffed a lot of times, and it can be very
stressful and frustrating, I still love my work. I wouldn't give it up for
anything in the world. I wouldn't. I love my work.*

*The majority of my residents are very grateful and they're very
thankful, very appreciative. Only a few, I would say, aren't. Every
now and then, perhaps someone will come, like the supervisors will
say, "You did a great job" or whatever. But you're not always appreci-
ated. You're not.*

*It can be really difficult at times. Because you're dealing with so
many people. Not just your residents, not just your co-workers, but
their families, social service, even dietary, people from activities. It's
very involved.*

*One time I went in to my resident to greet her and she told me that
she had had an encounter with this nursing assistant on the 11:00
P.M.–7:00 A.M. shift. And she told me that she had had an accident and
she called the nursing assistant—rang the buzzer—the resident was
incontinent of feces. You now what the nursing assistant told her to
do? Told her to clean it up herself! When she told me that, I was so
upset. Immediately, I went and informed the nurse and the nurse
informed the supervisor. She isn't here today. We don't need those
kinds of people here. We really don't. We need more dedicated people.
Like I told you before, there are a lot of people in this profession, but
only a few dedicated ones, only a few devoted ones that really love
their work. You really have to love* people. *You do. You have to love*
people *to do this kind of work. Because it's not easy. Everybody knows
it's not easy.*

Notes

1. Anthropology in an American Nursing Home

1. The Franklin Nursing Home and all other names of persons and places in this book are pseudonymns.

2. Background and Context

1. Skilled nursing care means twenty-four-hour inpatient skilled nursing, therapeutic, or restorative care.

2. Intermediate care I refers to twenty-four-hour inpatient preventive and supportive nursing services to patients with long-term or chronic illness or disability. These patients do not require treatments that must be administered under a registered nurse's or physician's supervision, but they do need help in the activities of daily living, such as dressing, bathing, eating, and walking. Intermediate care II refers to twenty-four-hour inpatient personal care and supervision for people who require minimal nursing-care needs. They are usually ambulatory, yet they may need assistance with activities of daily living from time to time.

3. These regulations vary state by state. For example, in a neighboring state an extra level of care is mandated for patients who need more care than skilled nursing care but less than would be necessary in an acute hospitalization episode. This one factor has several effects, such as providing greater state reimbursement to the long-term-care institution and reducing the number of resident hospitalizations.

4. The state census asks respondents their religion, but the United States census is prohibited by law from asking about religion directly. Therefore, estimates of the Jewish population derive either from determining the "Jewishness" of names or from assuming, as the United States census did, that Russian-born immigrants at the turn of the century were Jews.

3. Residents

1. Often people are admitted from the hospital with an acute infection producing temporary confusion. Sometimes the emotional upheaval of deciding to enter the nursing home creates disorientation, which clears up weeks later after an appropriate adjustment to the nursing home has been made (but often after the label of dementia has been applied). It has become clear that other diseases often masquerade as dementia, depression being a prime example.

2. Another reason that actual admission has lagged far behind the application process is a long waiting list. There is no waiting list and there are some empty beds at the time of this writing.

4. Conflicting Worldviews: Home versus Hospital

1. Retsinas properly points out the misplaced nostalgia underlying the home-hospital conflict. For example, "the homey home did not offer smoke detectors, sprinkler systems" (1986:51), and other features now considered standard and vital.

2. The social and emotional withdrawal exemplified by these behaviors could be subsumed under Glascock and Feinman's (1981) "death-hastening behaviors."

3. As far as I know, no other traditional mourning procedures are carried on in the nursing home, such as lighting candles.

4. If the hospitalization exceeds the period of time specifically allowed by current Medicaid rules (which change), the resident may have to be technically discharged and then readmitted to the nursing home when the hospitalization ends. In most nursing homes, which do not have policies of reserving rooms, residents forfeit their places when they are hospitalized.

5. This observation has been noted in "helping" agencies such as mental health clinics (see, for example, Gubrium and Buckholdt 1982). In such constructions, the "real" versus "fictive" family centers often on who "really" cares for the patient.

6. This behavior is corroborated in the nursing-home literature as well (for example, Retsinas 1986, Henderson 1981).

5. The Total Institution

1. The following are examples: When a nursing assistant or an orderly must lift a resident, certain procedures must be followed, and medical coverage is provided if an injury occurs when the procedures were followed. When a staff member is injured from lifting a resident, a meeting is called to determine whether benefits are allowed. Regulations prescribing the proper way to lift residents are issued to protect the nursing home from the cost of sick leaves stemming from staff

injuries. But often staff members do not follow the correct procedures because they may be complicated or require the cooperation of another person. Other issues regard the timing of calling in sick and the problem of volunteers' performing better than the other workers. Finally, pay schedules underlie many, if not most, of the disputes mediated and protected by the union. A month-long strike occurred in the mid-eighties.

2. Coser refined Goffman's scheme by including the category of "greedy institutions," which are marked by a seeming voluntariness of membership. Greedy institutions distinguish themselves from total institutions primarily by "maximizing assent to their styles of life by appearing highly desirable to the participants" (1974:6). Because greedy institutions require exclusive commitments, their members are usually powerless and propertyless and thus lack alternatives. Franklin fits the characterization because many of the residents speak of their free decision to enter. From the circumstances of their admissions, however, it is clear that the alternatives to nursing-home admission were limited. Central to the discussion of free will, therefore, is the availability to each individual of other social resources in the community.

3. In this context it is useful to note the contributions of Barton (1976) and Vail (1966) on the deleterious effects of institutionalization on inmates. Vail's book contains checklists for use by mental hospital personnel observing inmates to ensure that dehumanization is minimized. Barton describes "institutional neurosis" as a disease characterized by apathy, submissiveness, deterioration in personal habits, and a loss of individuality. He described a characteristic gait that accompanied this neurosis. He attributed these traits to the loss of contact with the outside, enforced idleness, staff behaviors, and lack of prospects. First published in 1959, Barton's book predated Goffman's *Asylums*.

4. These are "institutions established to care for persons felt to be both incapable and harmless; these are the homes for the blind, the aged, the orphaned, and the indigent. Second, there are places established to care for persons felt to be both incapable of looking after themselves and a threat to the community, albeit an unintended one: TB sanitaria, mental hospitals, and leprosaria. A third type of total institution is organized to protect the community against what are felt to be intentional dangers to it, with the welfare of the persons thus sequestered not the immediate issue: jails, penitentiaries, P.O.W. camps, and concentration camps. Fourth, there are institutions purportedly established the better to pursue some worklike task and justifying themselves only on these instrumental grounds: army barracks, ships, boarding schools, work camps, colonial compounds, and large mansions from the point of view of those who live in the servants' quarters. Finally, there are those establishments designed as retreats from the world even while often serving also as training stations for the religious; examples are abbeys, monasteries, convents, and other cloisters. This classification of total institutions is not neat, exhaustive, nor of immediate analytical use, but it does provide a purely denotative definition of the category as a concrete starting point" (1961:4–5).

6. Bridges to the Community

1. I encountered ambivalent reactions to my study at times. Will the research create tangible results? In various ways I heard about the "inferiority complex" of the nursing home in relation to the medical school and hospital.

2. A recent development at Franklin since fieldwork ended is that several community physicians now treat all the residents. This change does not totally eliminate the problems described here, however.

Another alternative that has been tried is the creation of a medical clinic in the nursing home. Instead of the physician's arriving unannounced, the physician would be available at the clinic by appointment. The physician would commit a certain block of time in which to examine residents. A resident would in turn go to the clinic for an appointment rather than traveling within the city to the individual doctor's office.

3. Physician visits range from once every two months for intermediate care II residents to once every thirty days for skilled-nursing-care residents.

4. When there was a strike, however, community volunteers were numerous and devoted. The crisis brought the nursing home and the community closer to each other.

5. In any one month, the rabbi might officiate at one Friday night service. The cantor might lead another Friday night service, and perhaps the sisterhood or another congregational committee would lead the other services. On average, rabbis have come to the nursing home since this plan was begun approximately once a month, though some rabbis have come more frequently.

6. Some rabbis attribute this reluctance to human nature. It is a rare individual who has the emotional and personal strength to confront his own mortality and fears by becoming personally involved in a nursing home or in any other place where the dying are housed. A similar reluctance is encountered on oncology wards. The desire to be financially helpful while maintaining a personal distance may reflect a common human trait.

7. Separation and Adaptation: The Passage

1. Although there is the quality of demotion, the differences are these: in Goffman's characterization of institutionalized individuals, being an inmate is like being demoted in an age-grade, but the demotion is temporary because the person is usually reinstated in society. In institutions other than jails or mental hospitals, the person returns to society at a higher status than when he left it. In his analysis of degradation ceremonies, Garfinkle referred primarily to people who are publicly denounced by their group and "remade" according to the new identity of the denounced person.

2. Conflicting information is often obtained. Social-service staff often find discrepancies regarding the financial status of the applicant. These discrepancies arise because of ignorance (due to, for example, misinformation, confusion about

Social Security, Medicare and Medicaid policies, death of a spouse who knew all the information, reluctance of the applicant or the family to admit to either a lower income or a higher one in order to save money for inheritance or to spare the family from being burdened or to be eligible for public monies dishonestly, to cite a few reasons), and various other intricate family dynamics. One staff member commented that the main problem in these families concerns money. Adult children dispute financial responsibility for their parents. Though there are no Medicare and Medicaid requirements binding children to pay for their parents' nursing-home care, Franklin needs as much private money as it can obtain. Sometimes the failing health of an aged parent is a major test of the solidarity of the family unit. Other misinformation results from incomplete medical records. The head trauma suffered twenty years ago, for example, may yield information regarding the applicant's present mental confusion, but the hospital records may be missing, and the physician may have moved, retired, or died. Depending on the particular family and the covert or overt reasons for seeking admission, family members may give incomplete or distorted information. The mother may have been punitive to her children while they were growing up, for example, and now that she lives alone and has many dependencies, the children may have difficulty in separating their own feelings toward her and each other vis-à-vis making realistic plans for her care. Small discrepancies in record keeping are commonplace. Place and date of birth information may not be known. The father, for example, may have used a certain date of birth for military service or other reasons; therefore, certain official documents show different dates.

3. Those residents who are able to go to the polls in the nursing home's district are taken there, whereas those residents who must remain on the premises are given the opportunity to use absentee ballots.

4. Researchers corroborate the importance of things that Franklin residents talked about to me. Things carry emotional significance and aid people in relocating (Kalymun 1983, Csikszentimihalyi and Rochberg-Halton 1981); carefully chosen items function as transitional objects in helping people feel "at home" (Schmitt, Redondo, and Wapner 1977).

5. An administrator stated that the issue has almost never come up in recent years. It follows that a person requesting admission to the nursing home is not well enough to drive.

6. To qualify for Medicaid assistance in this state at this writing, one needs to demonstrate medical need, first of all, and also have no more than four thousand dollars in liquid assets and four thousand dollars in life insurance. If the nursing-home resident is unmarried and has property, the property is sold and the proceeds go toward the payment of care. If there is a spouse, the property does not have to be sold. Currently, too, the new "50 percent ruling" allows that joint bank accounts do not have to be depleted when either the husband or the wife enters the nursing home, but the spouse who remains in the community can keep 50 percent of the bank account. Until recently, the joint bank account would have to be depleted to four thousand dollars before the spouse could qualify for Medicaid. Another new ruling is that a person is prohibited from qualifying for Medicaid if

he has disposed of his assets less than twenty-four months before admission. Medicaid pays approximately $20.00 less per day per resident than Franklin spends. Currently (fiscal 1987), the reimbursement from Medicaid is $56.50, and the cost per day per resident is $78.00. Though reimbursement rates were slightly less in the early 1980s when my fieldwork was taking place, the gap between reimbursement and cost per resident was approximately the same.

7. Because a large segment of this nursing-home population is incontinent, and even though the nursing home is clean, these smells are not uncommon.

8. The Limits of Exchange

1. Goodell (1985) distinguishes paternalism, patronage, and potlatch by their effects on the cohesion of the group. Her analysis of paternalism is similar to the argument offered here: autonomy and solidarity are undermined by the ideology inherent in the unreciprocated "gift."

2. Hazan (1980) does not make a similar claim in his work on elderly London Jews, however.

3. Years before fieldwork began, some Franklin residents did work for a local jewelry company for a time.

4. The differences between the sephardic nursing home and Franklin can be summed up as follows: (1) in the sephardic home most of the residents knew each other, (2) there was little if any stigma attached to entering the home, (3) residents had control and decision-making abilities, (4) volunteers from the community were very involved, and (5) the nursing-home population was healthier. Hendel-Sebestyen commented that because the nursing-home population was becoming more heterogeneous and sicker, she doubted that the same kind of community formation within the nursing home would continue as before.

5. Since fieldwork has ended, another discussion group has been organized by two volunteers at Franklin. Though various subjects are covered, the leaders have steered discussion from negative and disturbing topics, at times to the dismay of the residents (Lieberman 1988).

9. Liminality in the Nursing Home: The Endless Transition

1. Years ago, however, a past administrator at Franklin insisted that telephones be installed in the nursing home for the explicit purpose of reducing the separation of the institution from Harrison. Approximately one-third of the residents have telephones.

2. One of the changes discussed during my fieldwork concerned the duties of the night nursing shift. The administration was considering having the night shift initiate the resident wake-up procedures before leaving at 7:00 A.M. The daytime shift personnel sometimes complain that they have too many duties at the beginning of their shift. In this way timing is related to administrative and employee negotiations rather than to the needs of the residents.

3. Goldfarb (1965) has argued that the dependency of the elderly should not be labeled "regression," "second childhood," or evidence of "role reversal." Instead, he claims that lifelong dependency needs reassert themselves at certain times of the life cycle and are not related to these other concepts. Kalish (1967) notes that children and old people wish for an independence they do not have. Old people's dependency should be allowed without punishment, and the opportunity to be independent should be fostered. In a similar vein, Brody (1977) has maintained that throughout the life cycle there is a constant interdependence among people of different generations. She agrees that labels such as "regression," "second childhood," and "role reversal" are inappropriate. Because there are no normative standards for the dependency that old people exhibit, as there are for children, the dependency is considered illegitimate. She distinguishes actions that meet dependency needs from those that foster them. Marlowe (1973) conducted a study on this issue. Old people were separated into two groups. One group had their needs met, but they were not coddled. Continuity from the past was encouraged, autonomy was encouraged, access to the community was fostered, deviance was little tolerated, social interaction was encouraged, passivity was discouraged, and the residents were treated with warmth. The opposite was done in the second group, and negative results were found. This study was conducted when institutionalized elderly had to be relocated in other facilities. The "dependency-fostering environments" were associated with trauma and decline in residents' functioning as opposed to the contrasting environment.

4. Researchers (Henry 1963, Gresham 1976, Kayser-Jones 1981, Hazan 1980, Bennett 1963, Vail 1966, Barton 1976) have noted the infantilization and dehumanization of the elderly that occurs in nursing homes. Treating the residents as if they were all the same is one component of infantilizing behavior.

5. Gresham (1976) has indicated that the aged regress because they have learned that regression is the accepted way to obtain what they want.

6. Whenever I was present while this question was asked, it was asked discreetly.

7. Residents' roles in decision making at Franklin may be changing at this writing, as the institution incorporates a policy on patient procedures and treatment plans.

8. Some Jewish events are held in the nursing home: there are special holiday dinners, to which family members are invited; occasionally Jewish films are shown. One volunteer offered a program of Jewish films relating to Jewish identity. Though she tried to stimulate discussion of the issues, there was little response by the residents. In this example, as in others, whether the residents are competent to do more is difficult to discern.

9. Yiddish was taught to some staff members years before fieldwork took place. The staff member who related this information to me said that the course was thoroughly enjoyed.

10. Greene (1980) has shown that death anxiety among social workers was found to be significantly higher among those who worked with geriatric patients than among those who did not. Furthermore, death anxiety, as measured by Greene's scales, increased the longer the social workers stayed in the geriatric

field. Other research has documented similar relationships between a fear and avoidance of death and dying among those who are directly involved with people who are dying. Fleming and Brown (1981, 1983) and Gunter (1971) have noted nurses' feelings of inadequacy toward dying patients, their heightened death anxiety, their reluctance to talk about death with dying patients, and their emotional withdrawal from dying patients. Spence et al. (1968) related adverse medical student attitudes toward the geriatric patient. Gillis (1973) showed how the length of time that nurses spent working with elderly decreased their positive attitudes toward them. Townsend (1971) postulated that the anxiety of being with aged persons led to their treating them like children.

10. Summary and Conclusion

1. The recent introduction of the discussion group since fieldwork ended may be aiding the formation of community among certain residents (Lieberman 1988).

References

Agar, Michael. 1980. *The Professional Stranger: An Informal Introduction to Ethnography.* New York: Academic Press.

Amoss, Pamela T. 1981. Cultural Centrality and Prestige for the Elderly: The Coast Salish Case. In Christine L. Fry and contributors.

Amoss, Pamela T., and Stevan Harrell, eds. 1981. *Other Ways of Growing Old: Anthropological Perspectives.* Stanford: Stanford University Press.

Aronson, Stanley M., and Renée R. Shield. 1982. The Domain of the Elderly. *Rhode Island Medical Journal* 65:359–363.

Ball, Robert M. 1977. United States Policy toward the Elderly. In A. N. Exton-Smith and J. Grimley Evans, eds.

Barney, Jane L. 1987. Community Presence in Nursing Homes. *Gerontologist* 27:367–369.

Barton, Russell. 1976. *Institutional Neurosis.* Bristol: Wright. 1st pub. 1959.

Beauvoir, Simone de. 1972. *The Coming of Age.* New York: Warner Books.

Bellah, Robert N., Richard Madsen, William M. Sullivan, Ann Swidler, and Steven M. Tipton. 1985. *Habits of the Heart: Individualism and Commitment in American Life.* Berkeley: University of California Press.

Bennett, Ruth. 1963. The Meaning of Institutional Life. *Gerontologist* 3:117–123.

Bensman, Joseph, and Arthur J. Vidich. 1971. *The New American Society: The Revolution of the Middle Class.* Chicago: Quadrangle Books.

Berman, Rochel U., Audrey S. Weiner, and Gella S. Fishman. 1986. Yiddish: It's More Than a Language: In-service Training for Staff of a Jewish Home for the Aged. *Journal of Jewish Communal Service* 62 (4):328–334.

Birren, James E., and K. Warner Schaie, eds. 1977. *Handbook of the Psychology of Aging.* New York: Van Nostrand Reinhold.

Brody, Elaine M. 1977. Environmental Factors in Dependency. In A. N. Exton-Smith and J. Grimley Evans, eds.

——. 1985. Parent Care as a Normative Family Stress. *Gerontologist* 25:19–29.

References

Butler, Robert N. 1975. *Why Survive? Being Old in America.* New York: Harper and Row.

Clark, M. Margaret. 1973. Contributions of Cultural Anthropology to the Study of the Aged. In Laura Nader and Thomas W. Maretzki, eds.

Clinton, Robert, Renée Rose Shield, and Stanley M. Aronson. 1983. Patterns of Survival in a Home for the Aged. Paper presented at the Northeast Gerontological Society annual meeting, Newport, R.I.

Cool, Linda. 1980. Ethnicity and Aging: Continuity through Change for Elderly Corsicans. In Christine L. Fry and contributors.

Coser, Lewis A. 1974. *Greedy Institutions: Patterns of Undivided Commitment.* New York: Free Press.

Csikszentmihalyi, Mihaly, and Eugene Rochberg-Halton. 1981. *The Meaning of Things: Domestic Symbols and the Self.* New York: Cambridge University Press.

Cumming, Elaine, and William Henry. 1961. *Growing Old: The Process of Disengagement.* New York: Basic Books.

Douglas, Mary. 1966. *Purity and Danger: An Analysis of Concepts of Pollution and Taboo.* London: Routledge and Kegan Paul.

Dowd, James P. 1975. Aging as Exchange: A Preface to Theory. *J of Gerontology* 30:584–594.

Estes, Carroll. 1979. *The Aging Enterprise: A Critical Examination of Social Policies and Services for the Aged.* San Francisco: Jossey-Bass Publishers.

Exton-Smith, A. N., and J. Grimley Evans, eds. 1977. *Care of the Elderly: Meeting the Challenge of Dependency.* New York: Grune and Stratton.

Faulwell, Margaret, and Rhoda S. Pomerantz. 1981. Physician Influence in the Selection of Institutionalization of the Elderly. In Christine L. Fry and contributors.

Fishbein, Carol Farb, and Pamela Kaitin-Miller. 1986. Residents' Preferences for Management of Death in a Nursing Home. Unpub. MSW project, Rhode Island College.

Fleming, Stephen, and Isabel Brown. 1981. Nurses' Educational and Personal Preparation in Caring for the Dying. Unpub. ms.

——. 1983. The Impact of a Death Eduation Program for Nurses in a Long-Term Care Hospital. *Gerontologist* 23:192–195.

Foner, Anne, and David I. Kertzer. 1978. Transitions over the Life-Course: Lessons from Age-Set Societies. *American Journal of Sociology* 83:1081–1104.

Foner, Nancy. 1984. *Ages in Conflict: A Cross-Cultural Perspective on Inequality between Old and Young.* New York: Columbia University Press.

Fretwell, Marsha. 1982. Personal communication.

Freymann, John Gordon. 1974. *The American Health Care System: Its Genesis and Trajectory.* Baltimore: Williams and Wilkins.

Fry, Christine L., and contributors. 1980. *Aging in Culture and Society: Comparative Viewpoints and Strategies.* New York: Bergin.

Fry, Christine L., and contributors. 1981. *Dimensions: Aging, Culture, and Health.* New York: Bergin.

Garfinkle, Harold. 1956. Conditions of Successful Degradation Ceremonies. *American Journal of Sociology* 61:420–424.

Gennep, Arnold van. 1960. *The Rites of Passage.* Chicago: University of Chicago Press. 1st pub. 1908.

Gillis, Sr. Marion. 1973. Attitudes of Nursing Personnel toward the Aged. *Nursing Research* 22:517–520.

Glascock, Anthony P., and Susan L. Feinman. 1981. Social Asset or Social Burden: Treatment of the Aged in Non-industrial Societies. In Christine L. Fry and contributors.

Goffman, Erving. 1959. *The Presentation of Self in Everyday Life.* New York: Doubleday.

———. 1961. *Asylums.* New York: Doubleday.

Goldfarb, Alvin I. 1965. Psychodynamics and the Three-Generation Family. In Ethel Shanas and Gordon F. Streib, eds.

Goldstein, Sidney. 1981. Jews in the United States: Perspectives from Demography. *American Jewish Year Book,* 3–59. Philadelphia: Jewish Publication Society.

Goldstein, Sidney, and Calvin Goldscheider. 1968. *Jewish Americans: Three Generations in a Jewish Community.* Englewood Cliffs, N.J.: Prentice-Hall.

Goodell, Grace E. 1985. Paternalism, Patronage, and Potlatch: The Dynamics of Giving and Being Given To. *Current Anthropology.* 26:247–266.

Greene, Roberta Rubin. 1980. Ageism and Death Anxiety as Related to Geriatric Social Work as a Career Choice. Unpub. Ph.D. diss., University of Maryland School of Social Work.

Gresham, M. L. 1976. The Infantilization of the Elderly: A Developing Concept. *Nursing Forum* 15:195–210.

Gubrium, Jaber F. 1975. *Living and Dying at Murray Manor.* New York: St. Martin's Press.

Gubrium, Jaber F., ed. 1976. *Time, Roles, and Self in Old Age.* New York: Human Sciences Press.

Gubrium, Jaber F., and David R. Buckholdt. 1982. Fictive Family: Everyday Usage, Analytic, and Human Service Considerations. *American Anthropologist* 84:878–885.

Gulliver, P. H. 1963. *Social Control in an African Society.* London: Routledge and Kegan Paul.

Gunter, Laurie M. 1971. Students' Attitudes toward Geriatric Nursing. *Nursing Outlook* 19:466–469.

Gutmann, David. 1976. Alternatives to Disengagement: The Old Man of the Highland Druze. In J. F. Gubrium, ed.

———. 1977. The Cross-Cultural Perspective: Notes toward a Comparative Psychology of Aging. In James E. Birren and K. Warner Schaie, eds.

References

Hazan, Haim. 1980. *The Limbo People: A Study of the Constitution of the Time Universe among the Aged.* Boston: Routledge and Kegan Paul.

———. 1984. Continuity and Transformation among the Aged: A Study in the Anthropology of Time. *Current Anthropology* 25:567–578.

Hendel-Sebestyen, Giselle. 1969. The Sephardic Home: Ethnic Homogeneity and Cultural Traditions in a Total Institution. Unpub. Ph.D. diss., Columbia University.

———. 1979. Role Diversity: Toward the Development of Community in a Total Institutional Setting. In Jennie Keith, ed.

Henderson, Joseph Neil. 1981. Nursing Home Housekeepers: Indigenous Agents of Psychosocial Support. *Human Organization* 40:300–305.

Henry, Jules. 1963. *Culture against Man.* New York: Random House.

Hochschild, Arlie Russell. 1973. *The Unexpected Community: Portrait of an Old Age Subculture.* Berkeley: University of California Press.

Howell, S. 1976. Recent Advances in Studies of Physical Environments of the Elderly. Talk presented at the Environmental Psychology Program, CUNY Graduate Center, New York.

Howsden, Jackie L. 1981. *Work and the Helpless Self.* Washington, D.C.: University Press of America.

James, Alice, W. L. James, and H. L. Smith. 1984. Reciprocity as a Coping Strategy of the Elderly: A Rural Irish Perspective. *Gerontologist* 24:483–489.

Kalish, Richard A. 1967. Of Children and Grandfathers: A Speculative Essay on Dependency. *Gerontologist* 7:65–69, 79.

Kalymun, Mary. 1983. Factors Influencing Elderly Women's Decisions Concerning Living-Room Possessions during Relocation. Paper presented at the Environmental Design Research Association, University of Nebraska, Lincoln.

Kayser-Jones, Jeanie Schmit. 1981. *Old, Alone, and Neglected: Care of the Aged in Scotland and the United States.* Berkeley: University of California Press.

Keith, Jennie. 1979. The Ethnography of Old Age. *Anthropological Quarterly* (special issue) 52.

———. 1982a. *Old People as People: Social and Cultural Influences on Aging and Old Age.* Boston: Little, Brown.

———. 1982b. *Old People, New Lives: Community Creation in a Retirement Residence.* Chicago: University of Chicago Press. (Orig. Jennie-Keith Ross). Orig. pub. 1977.

Kronenberg, Irving. 1983. Bereavement Research and Intervention in a Long Term Care Setting. Paper presented at the Northeast Gerontological Society Meeting, Newport, R.I.

———. 1984. Personal communication.

Laird, Carobeth. 1979. *Limbo.* Novato, Calif.: Chandler and Sharp.

Lappin, Lynn Fuldauer, and Rhonda Speert Grossman. 1982. Loosening the Tie That Binds: Residents in Long-Term Care and Their Families. *Journal of Jewish Communal Service* 58:343–349.

Leaf, Alexander. 1973. Getting Old. *Scientific American* 22:45–52.

——. 1982. Aging, Longevity, Prevention, and Cure: Our Professional Futures. *Rhode Island Medical Journal* 65:365–369.

Legesse, Asmaron. 1979. Age Sets and Retirement Communities: Comparison and Comment. In Jennie Keith, ed.

Lévi-Strauss, Claude. 1949. *The Elementary Structures of Kinship.* Boston: Beacon Press. 1965 ed.

Lieberman, M. 1973. Grouchiness: A Survival Asset. *University of Chicago Alumni Magazine,* April:11–14.

Lieberman, Morton A., and Sheldon Tobin. 1983. *The Experience of Old Age: Stress, Coping, and Survival.* New York: Basic Books.

Lieberman, Seth. 1988. Jewish Life in Old Age: Forming, Unforming and Transforming Communal Ties. Unpub. ms.

Linzer, Norman. 1986. The Obligations of Adult Children to Aged Parents: A View from Jewish Tradition. *Journal of Aging and Judaism* 1:34–48.

Liu, Korbin, and Kenneth G. Manton. 1983. The Characteristics and Utilization Pattern of an Admission Cohort of Nursing Home Patients. *Gerontologist* 23:92–98.

——. 1984. The Characteristics and Utilization Pattern of an Admission Cohort of Nursing Home Patients (II). *Gerontologist* 24:70–76.

Mace, Nancy L., and Peter V. Rabins. 1981. *The 36-Hour Day: A Family Guide to Caring for Persons with Alzheimer's Disease, Related Dementing Illness, and Memory Loss in Later Life.* Baltimore: Johns Hopkins University Press.

Marlowe, R. A. 1973. Effects of Environment on Elderly State Hospital Relocators. In *44th Annual Meeting of the Pacific Sociological Association.* Scottsdale, Ariz. Mimeo.

Mauss, Marcel. 1925. *The Gift: Forms and Functions of Exchange in Archaic Societies.* New York: Norton. 1967 ed.

Michel, Sonya. 1977. Children, Institutions, and Community: The Jewish Orphanage of Rhode Island, 1909–1942. *Rhode Island Jewish Historical Notes* 7 (3):385–400.

Mitchell, Janet B. 1982. Physician Visits to Nursing Homes. *Gerontologist* 22:45–48.

Mitchell, Janet B., and Helene T. Hewes. 1986. Why Won't Physicians Make Nursing Home Visits? *Gerontologist* 26:650–654.

Moore, Sally Falk. 1978. Old Age in a Life-Term Social Arena. In Barbara G. Myerhoff and Andrei Simič, eds.

Murphy, Robert F. 1987. *The Body Silent.* New York: Henry Holt.

Myerhoff, Barbara G. 1978. A Symbol Perfected in Death. In Barbara G. Myerhoff and Andrei Simič, eds.

——. 1979. *Number Our Days.* New York: E. P. Dutton.

——. 1982. Rites of Passage: Process and Paradox. In Victor Turner, ed.

Myerhoff, Barbara G., and Andrei Simič, eds. 1978. *Life's Career-Aging: Cultural Variations on Growing Old.* Beverly Hills: Sage Publications.

Nader, Laura, and Thomas W. Maretzki, eds. 1973. *Cultural Illness and Health.* Washington, D.C.: American Anthropological Association.

References

National Center for Health Statistics. 1979. *The National Nursing Home Survey: 1977 Summary for the United States.* Vital and Health Statistics, Series 13, No. 43. DHEW Pub. No. (PHS) 79-1794.

Neugarten, Bernice L., ed. 1968. *Middle Age and Aging.* Chicago: University of Chicago.

————. 1979. The Young-Old . . . A New North American Phenomenon. In Couchiching Institute on Public Affairs. Toronto: Couchiching Institute on Public Affairs.

Nydegger, Corinne. 1983. Family Ties of the Aged in Cross-Cultural Perspective. *Gerontologist* 23:26–32.

Palmore, Erdman. 1975. The Honorable Elders: A Cross-Cultural Analysis of Aging in Japan. Durham: Duke University Press.

Retsinas, Joan. 1986. *It's OK, Mom: The Nursing Home from a Sociological Perspective.* New York: Tiresias Press.

Rosenwaike, Ira. 1986. The American Jewish Elderly in Transition. *Journal of Jewish Communal Service* 62 (4):283–291.

Rosenwaike, Ira, and Arthur Dolinsky. 1987. The Changing Demographic Determinants of the Growth of the Extreme Aged. *Gerontologist* 27:275–280.

Rouslin, Marcia. 1981. Playing Musical Chairs with Elderly Skilled Patients: Medicare, Medicaid Regulations. Unpub. ms.

Schmitt, V., J. P. Redondo, and S. Wapner. 1977. The Role of Transitional Objects in Adult Adaptation. Unpub. ms.

Shanas, Ethel. 1979. Social Myth as Hypothesis: The Case of the Family Life of Old People. *Gerontologist* 19:3–9.

Shanas, Ethel, and Gordon F. Streib, eds. 1965. *Social Structure and the Family: Generational Relationships.* Englewood Cliffs, N.J.: Prentice-Hall.

Shore, David, Carol A. Overman, and Richard Jed Wyatt. 1983. Improving Accuracy in the Diagnosis of Alzheimer's Disease. *Journal of Clinical Psychiatry* 44 (6):207–212.

Siegel, Jacob S. 1978. *Demographic Aspects of Aging and the Older Population in the United States. Current Population Reports.* Special Studies, Series P-23, No. 59. Washington, D.C.: United States Bureau of the Census.

Smolar, Leivy. 1985. Context and Text: Realities and Jewish Perspectives on the Aged. Journal of Jewish Communal Service 62 (1):1–7.

Sokolovsky, Jay, and Carl Cohen. 1981. Being Old in the Inner City: Support Systems of the SRO Aged. In Christine L. Fry and contributors.

Spence, Donald L., E. M. Feigenbaum, Faith Fitzgerald, and Janet Roth. 1968. Medical Student Attitudes towards the Geriatric Patient. *Journal of the Amer Geriatrics Society* 16:976–983.

Steinberg, Alan, L. Jaime Fitten, and Norman Kachuck. 1986. Patient Participation in Treatment Decision-making in the Nursing Home: The Issue of Competence. *Gerontologist* 26:362–366.

Thomas, William C., Jr. 1969. *Nursing Homes and Public Policy: Drift and Decision in New York State.* Ithaca: Cornell University Press.

Townsend, Claire. 1971. *Old Age: The Last Segregation*. Ralph Nader's Study Group Report on Nursing Homes. New York: Grossman Publishers.

Turner, Victor. 1967. *The Forest of Symbols*. Ithaca: Cornell University Press.

——. 1968. *The Drums of Affliction*. Reprint, Ithaca: Cornell University Press, 1981.

——. 1969. *The Ritual Process*. Reprint, Ithaca: Cornell University Press, 1977.

——. 1974. *Dramas, Fields, and Metaphors*. Ithaca: Cornell University Press.

——, ed. 1982. *Celebration: Studies in Festivity and Ritual*. Washington, D.C.: Smithsonian Institution Press.

——. 1982. *From Ritual to Theatre: The Human Seriousness of Play*. New York: Performing Arts Journal Publications.

Updike, John. 1958. *The Poorhouse Fair*. New York: Knopf.

Vail, David J. 1966. *Dehumanization and the Institutional Career*. Springfield, Ill.: Charles C. Thomas.

Vatuk, Sylvia. 1980. Withdrawal and Disengagement as a Cultural Response to Aging in India. In Christine L. Fry and contributors.

Vladeck, Bruce C. 1980. *Unloving Care: The Nursing Home Tragedy*. New York: Basic Books.

Wax, M. 1962. The Changing Role of the Home for the Aged. *Gerontologist* 2:128–133.

Weber, Max. 1947. *The Theory of Social and Economic Organization*. Trans. and ed. Talcott Parsons. New York: Oxford University Press.

Weinberg, Jack. 1976. On Adding Insight to Injury. *Gerontologist* 16:4–10.

Wilson, Barbara. 1983. Personal communication.

Windley, P. G., and G. Ernst, eds. 1975. *Theory Development in Environment and Aging*. Washington, D.C.: Gerontological Society.

Wingard, Deborah L., Denise Williams Jones, and Robert M. Kaplan. 1987. Institutional Care Utilization by the Elderly. A Critical Review. *Gerontologist* 27:156–163.

Index

Administration, 93, 101
Admission, nursing-home, 42–43, 53; process, 46, 126–130, 228–229; reasons for, 33, 43, 45–46, 126–128; timing of, 128, 226; trauma of, 129–131, 226
Alzheimer's disease (SDAT). See Dementia.
Anthropology, cultural, 10–16; and aging, 12, 17–18; at home, 13–14
Anti-Semitism, 202–203
Anxiety, death, 231–232

Bickering, 170–171
Bureaucracy, 91–96

Cardio-pulmonary rescuscitation (CPR), 68
Care, levels of, 32, 34–35, 225; and room changes, 72–74
Chagga, 55, 204
Children, and dependency, 193; residents as, 22–23, 156–157, 194–200, 209. See also Infantilization.
Clark, M. Margaret, 193
Communitas, 22, 53, 124–126, 184; and lack of, 205–209, 214–216, 220
Community, feelings of, 19–20, 65, 78, 125; and bickering, 170–171; councils, 217. See also Communitas.

Death, anxiety about, 231–232; avoidance of subject, 22, 69; of children, 60, 204–205; as an enemy, 171; "hidden sui-

cide," 129, management of, 69–71; memorials for, 70–71, 205–207, 219; silence about, 205–206; timing of, 191–192, 204–205
Dementia, demented persons, 43–44, 135, 226; avoidance of, 56; behavior of, 137–138; and room changes, 74; sounds of, 136
Dependency, 22–23, 98, 128, 215; and decision-making, 199–200, 216–217; expectation of, 176, 231; in liminality, 192–194; ratios, 28; and reciprocity, 153–154, 157. See also Rites of passage.
Douglas, Mary, 120–121

Elderly, demography of, 28–29
Exchange. See Reciprocity.

Families. See Residents, Franklin.
Fieldwork, anthropological, 16–19
Food, 65, 95; mix-ups of, 139; significance of, 134–135
Friendships and reciprocity, 155–156, 166; between residents and staff, 74–76, 173–174

Gennep, Arnold van, 21
Goffman, Erving, 20–21, 91, 197, 214, 227–228; theory of, 96–104
Goldfarb mental status test, 44
Gubrium, Jaber F., 66; and "alertness cliques," 56; "breaking up" a home,

Gubrium, Jaber F. (cont.)
132–133; and passing time, 185–186; and routine, 189; and "supporters," 164; and talk, 167; and wristbands, 99

Hazan, Haim, 168, 192, 195, 201–202
Hendel-Sebestyen, Giselle, 157, 230
Hochschild, Arlie Russell, 191, 205–208
Hospice, 71, 205

Individualism, 161
Infantilization, 16, 20; residents as children, 194–200, 209. See also Children; Dependency.
Institutions, greedy, 227
Institutions, total, 20–21, 91, 96–104; and children, 185; description of, 227; and work, 158

Jews, Jewish, 18–20; in community, 22, 33–34, 59–60, 118–119, 201–202; ritual, 20, 205–209; scripture on aging, 163; staff, 37, 67–68. See also Religion.

Kayser-Jones, Jeanie Schmit, 156, 172, 194–195
Keith, Jennie, 206–208

Liminality, 21–24, 53, 65, 183–209; as dangerous, 120, 124–125; institutionalization as, 103–104; and separation, 184–185; unresolved, 207–209, 214–216

Medicaid, Medicare, 32, 35, 115, 134, 156; qualifications for, 229–230; and room changes, 226
Merrill Court, 191, 205–208
Moore, Sally Falk, 55, 204
Murphy, Robert, 13, 77, 193
Murray Manor, 56, 66, 132–133, 164, 167, 185–186, 189
Myerhoff, Barbara G.: and children, 161–162; and female dominance, 58; and injury, 170–171; and rituals, 124–125, 218–219; and strategy of intimacy, 172; and witnessing, 55, 168

Nurses, Franklin, 35–36, 67–68, 70, 93–94; in relation to hospital, 117; versus

social workers, 67–69, 95–96
Nursing assistants, Franklin, 92–95; attitudes of, 69, 100; training of, 36
Nursing homes, funding of, 31–32; history of, 30–32; perception of, 23, 32; population of, 29–30; regulations of, 31–33; study of, 18, 24
Nursing pools, 36

Orderlies, Franklin, 35–36, 92–95

Participant-observation, 12, 19
Patients. See Residents, Franklin.
People-work, 100–101
Physical therapy, 76–79, 178, 207–208, 215–216
Physicians, 66, 68–70, 93–94; regularity of visits, 228; reluctance to visit nursing homes, 22, 115–116; residents' perceptions of, 116

Rabbis, 22, 119, 228
Reciprocity, and control, 156–160; and dependency, 153–154; and doing favors for, 134, 137, 158, 172–173; and friendship, 155–156; and individualism, 160–161; in Jewish scripture, 163; in kinship, 160–163; in rites of passage, 154–155, 207–209, 214–215; theory of, 21–23, 153–154; and work, 78
Religion, 200–204
Reminiscence, 166, 168
Residents, Franklin: ages of, 42–43; families of, 45–46, 53–54, 58–60, 160–163, 177–178, 190; Medicaid-reimbursed, 35; occupations of, 45, 54; origins of, 44–45, 54, 57; strategies of, 53–60, 98–99, 137–140, 164–179, 197–198
Restraints, physical, 67, 116
Rites of passage, 18, 21–23, 124, 140, 215; and dependency, 192–194; institutionalization as, 103–104, 184; and teaching, 124–125, 194
Ritual, 21–23, 65, 218–219; lack of, 22–24, 205–209, 216
Room changes, 72–74, 95

Senility. See Dementia.
Sex: perceived differences between men

Sex (*cont.*)
  and women, 57–58; ratios in Franklin
  population, 42–43; sexual behavior,
  198–199
Social Security, 31–32
Social workers, Franklin, 35–36, 70, 73,
  75; versus nurses, 67–69, 95–96
Strategies. *See* Residents, Franklin.
Strike, 59, 75–76, 92–93; and volunteers,
  228. *See also* Union, labor.

Talk, 20, 76–78, 165–166; bickering, 169–
  171; and linguistic "enders," 167; monitoring of, 165–166; by staff, 169; "talk-
  stop," 167–169; as trivial, 196–197; and
  witnessing, 168
Theft, 159

Things, acquisition of, 137; importance of,
  229; loss of, 132–135
Time, 185–192; of future peril, 191–192;
  and timelessness, 23, 101, 208–209
Touch, importance of, 178–179
Turner, Victor, 21; and liminality, 183–
  184, 207, 216; and rites of passage, 125

Union, labor, 35, 75–76, 92–93; issues of,
  226–227; and volunteers, 120

Volunteers, Franklin, 119–121; during
  strike, 228

Witnessing, 55, 168
Worldviews, 65–69, 79, 95, 101

Yiddish, 14, 201–202, 218, 231

Library of Congress Cataloging-in-Publication Data

Shield, Renée Rose.
  Uneasy endings.

  (Anthropology of contemporary issues)
  Bibliography: p.
  Includes index.
  1. Nursing homes—United States.   2. Nursing home patients—United
States.   I. Title.   II. Series.
RA997.S53   1988   362.1'6'0973   88-47743
ISBN 0-8014-2159-4 (alk. paper)
ISBN 0-8014-9490-7 (pbk. : alk. paper)